The Queens closet opened incomparable secrets in physick, chyrurgery, preserving, candying, and cookery, as they were presented unto the Queen by the most experienced persons of our times (1658)

W. M

The Queens closet opened incomparable secrets in physick, chyrurgery, preserving, candying, and cookery, as they were presented unto the Queen by the most experienced persons of our times
Queen's delight.
Art of preserving, conserving and candying.
W. M.
[Edition statement:] The fourth edition corrected, with many additions : together with three exact tables, one of them never before printed.
"The table" [i.e. index]: p. [1]-[23].
"The approvers names": prelim. p. [7]-[10].
Added t.p. on p. [193]: A queens delighgt [sic] or, The art of preserving, conserving, and candying, with imprint: London : Printed by R. Wood for Nath. Brooke, 1658.
[10], 300, [23] p.
London : Printed for Nathaniel Brooke,
Wing / M98
English
Reproduction of the original in the Bodleian Library

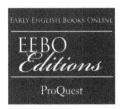

Early English Books Online (EEBO) Editions

Imagine holding history in your hands.

Now you can. Digitally preserved and previously accessible only through libraries as Early English Books Online, this rare material is now available in single print editions. Thousands of books written between 1475 and 1700 and ranging from religion to astronomy, medicine to music, can be delivered to your doorstep in individual volumes of high-quality historical reproductions.

We have been compiling these historic treasures for more than 70 years. Long before such a thing as "digital" even existed, ProQuest founder Eugene Power began the noble task of preserving the British Museum's collection on microfilm. He then sought out other rare and endangered titles, providing unparalleled access to these works and collaborating with the world's top academic institutions to make them widely available for the first time. This project furthers that original vision.

These texts have now made the full journey -- from their original printing-press versions available only in rare-book rooms to online library access to new single volumes made possible by the partnership between artifact preservation and modern printing technology. A portion of the proceeds from every book sold supports the libraries and institutions that made this collection possible, and that still work to preserve these invaluable treasures passed down through time.

This is history, traveling through time since the dawn of printing to your own personal library.

Initial Proquest EEBO Print Editions collections include:

Early Literature

This comprehensive collection begins with the famous Elizabethan Era that saw such literary giants as Chaucer, Shakespeare and Marlowe, as well as the introduction of the sonnet. Traveling through Jacobean and Restoration literature, the highlight of this series is the Pollard and Redgrave 1475-1640 selection of the rarest works from the English Renaissance.

Early Documents of World History

This collection combines early English perspectives on world history with documentation of Parliament records, royal decrees and military documents that reveal the delicate balance of Church and State in early English government. For social historians, almanacs and calendars offer insight into daily life of common citizens. This exhaustively complete series presents a thorough picture of history through the English Civil War.

Historical Almanacs

Historically, almanacs served a variety of purposes from the more practical, such as planting and harvesting crops and plotting nautical routes, to predicting the future through the movements of the stars. This collection provides a wide range of consecutive years of "almanacks" and calendars that depict a vast array of everyday life as it was several hundred years ago.

Early History of Astronomy & Space

Humankind has studied the skies for centuries, seeking to find our place in the universe. Some of the most important discoveries in the field of astronomy were made in these texts recorded by ancient stargazers, but almost as impactful were the perspectives of those who considered their discoveries to be heresy. Any independent astronomer will find this an invaluable collection of titles arguing the truth of the cosmic system.

Early History of Industry & Science

Acting as a kind of historical Wall Street, this collection of industry manuals and records explores the thriving industries of construction; textile, especially wool and linen; salt; livestock; and many more.

Early English Wit, Poetry & Satire

The power of literary device was never more in its prime than during this period of history, where a wide array of political and religious satire mocked the status quo and poetry called humankind to transcend the rigors of daily life through love, God or principle. This series comments on historical patterns of the human condition that are still visible today.

Early English Drama & Theatre

This collection needs no introduction, combining the works of some of the greatest canonical writers of all time, including many plays composed for royalty such as Queen Elizabeth I and King Edward VI. In addition, this series includes history and criticism of drama, as well as examinations of technique.

Early History of Travel & Geography

Offering a fascinating view into the perception of the world during the sixteenth and seventeenth centuries, this collection includes accounts of Columbus's discovery of the Americas and encompasses most of the Age of Discovery, during which Europeans and their descendants intensively explored and mapped the world. This series is a wealth of information from some the most groundbreaking explorers.

Early Fables & Fairy Tales

This series includes many translations, some illustrated, of some of the most well-known mythologies of today, including Aesop's Fables and English fairy tales, as well as many Greek, Latin and even Oriental parables and criticism and interpretation on the subject.

Early Documents of Language & Linguistics

The evolution of English and foreign languages is documented in these original texts studying and recording early philology from the study of a variety of languages including Greek, Latin and Chinese, as well as multilingual volumes, to current slang and obscure words. Translations from Latin, Hebrew and Aramaic, grammar treatises and even dictionaries and guides to translation make this collection rich in cultures from around the world.

Early History of the Law

With extensive collections of land tenure and business law "forms" in Great Britain, this is a comprehensive resource for all kinds of early English legal precedents from feudal to constitutional law, Jewish and Jesuit law, laws about public finance to food supply and forestry, and even "immoral conditions." An abundance of law dictionaries, philosophy and history and criticism completes this series.

Early History of Kings, Queens and Royalty

This collection includes debates on the divine right of kings, royal statutes and proclamations, and political ballads and songs as related to a number of English kings and queens, with notable concentrations on foreign rulers King Louis IX and King Louis XIV of France, and King Philip II of Spain. Writings on ancient rulers and royal tradition focus on Scottish and Roman kings, Cleopatra and the Biblical kings Nebuchadnezzar and Solomon.

Early History of Love, Marriage & Sex

Human relationships intrigued and baffled thinkers and writers well before the postmodern age of psychology and self-help. Now readers can access the insights and intricacies of Anglo-Saxon interactions in sex and love, marriage and politics, and the truth that lies somewhere in between action and thought.

Early History of Medicine, Health & Disease

This series includes fascinating studies on the human brain from as early as the 16th century, as well as early studies on the physiological effects of tobacco use. Anatomy texts, medical treatises and wound treatment are also discussed, revealing the exponential development of medical theory and practice over more than two hundred years.

Early History of Logic, Science and Math

The "hard sciences" developed exponentially during the 16th and 17th centuries, both relying upon centuries of tradition and adding to the foundation of modern application, as is evidenced by this extensive collection. This is a rich collection of practical mathematics as applied to business, carpentry and geography as well as explorations of mathematical instruments and arithmetic; logic and logicians such as Aristotle and Socrates; and a number of scientific disciplines from natural history to physics.

Early History of Military, War and Weaponry

Any professional or amateur student of war will thrill at the untold riches in this collection of war theory and practice in the early Western World. The Age of Discovery and Enlightenment was also a time of great political and religious unrest, revealed in accounts of conflicts such as the Wars of the Roses.

Early History of Food

This collection combines the commercial aspects of food handling, preservation and supply to the more specific aspects of canning and preserving, meat carving, brewing beer and even candy-making with fruits and flowers, with a large resource of cookery and recipe books. Not to be forgotten is a "the great eater of Kent," a study in food habits.

Early History of Religion

From the beginning of recorded history we have looked to the heavens for inspiration and guidance. In these early religious documents, sermons, and pamphlets, we see the spiritual impact on the lives of both royalty and the commoner. We also get insights into a clergy that was growing ever more powerful as a political force. This is one of the world's largest collections of religious works of this type, revealing much about our interpretation of the modern church and spirituality.

Early Social Customs

Social customs, human interaction and leisure are the driving force of any culture. These unique and quirky works give us a glimpse of interesting aspects of day-to-day life as it existed in an earlier time. With books on games, sports, traditions, festivals, and hobbies it is one of the most fascinating collections in the series.

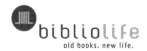

The BiblioLife Network

This project was made possible in part by the BiblioLife Network (BLN), a project aimed at addressing some of the huge challenges facing book preservationists around the world. The BLN includes libraries, library networks, archives, subject matter experts, online communities and library service providers. We believe every book ever published should be available as a high-quality print reproduction; printed on-demand anywhere in the world. This insures the ongoing accessibility of the content and helps generate sustainable revenue for the libraries and organizations that work to preserve these important materials.

The following book is in the "public domain" and represents an authentic reproduction of the text as printed by the original publisher. While we have attempted to accurately maintain the integrity of the original work, there are sometimes problems with the original work or the micro-film from which the books were digitized. This can result in minor errors in reproduction. Possible imperfections include missing and blurred pages, poor pictures, markings and other reproduction issues beyond our control. Because this work is culturally important, we have made it available as part of our commitment to protecting, preserving, and promoting the world's literature.

GUIDE TO FOLD-OUTS MAPS and OVERSIZED IMAGES

The book you are reading was digitized from microfilm captured over the past thirty to forty years. Years after the creation of the original microfilm, the book was converted to digital files and made available in an online database.

In an online database, page images do not need to conform to the size restrictions found in a printed book. When converting these images back into a printed bound book, the page sizes are standardized in ways that maintain the detail of the original. For large images, such as fold-out maps, the original page image is split into two or more pages

Guidelines used to determine how to split the page image follows:

- Some images are split vertically; large images require vertical and horizontal splits.
- For horizontal splits, the content is split left to right.
- For vertical splits, the content is split from top to bottom.
- For both vertical and horizontal splits, the image is processed from top left to bottom right.

THE QUEENS CLOSET OPENED:

Incomparable Secrets in Physick, Chyrurgery, Preserving, Candying, and Cookery;

As they were presented unto the QUEEN

By the most Experienced Persons of our times, many whereof were honoured with her own Practise, when she pleased to descend to these more private Recreations.

The Fourth Edition corrected, with many Additions: together with three exact Tables, one of them never before Printed.

Transcribed from the true Copies of her MAJESTIES own Receipt Books, by W. M. one of her late Servants.

Vivit post funera Virtus

London, Printed for Nathaniel Brooks at the Angel in Cornhill, 1658.

+ Nyrghi
   Au xiii 1846

THE QUEENS CLOSET OPENED:

To those persons of Honour and Quality, that presented many of these admirable Receipts at the Feet of the Queens Majesty, the Publisher resigns them with his prostrate Service whilst he breathes, and is

W. M.

Generous Reader,

MY particular Relation for many years to Her Majesties service, might easily, should I write my own History, rid thee of all scruples touching the truth of this Collection, there being few or none of these Receipts presented to her Majesty,

The Epistle

jesty, which were not transcribed into her Book by my self, the Original papers being most of them preserved in my own hands, which I kept as so many Reliques, and should sooner have parted with my dearest blood, then to have suffered them to be publick. But since my Soveraign Mistress her banishment, as also this continued change, being diffident of the alteration of these times, I could not deny the importunities of a person of Honour, to whom I was oblieged, who got a transcript of one of the true Copies from me, but by ill fortune, either lent or lost it; which I had never known from himself, but that to my no small amazement I found no less then two other Copies abroad; the sad consideration whereof inforced me to consult with my friends, who all of them advised me to dispatch my original copy to the Press to prevent those false ones; for otherwise I should not have thought it less then Sacriledge, had not the lock been first pickt, to have opened the Closet of my distressed Soveraign Mistress without her Royal Assent. But since that unfortunate miscarriage, I thought this publication to stand upon no ordinary tearms of honor, as it might con-

The Epistle.

continue my Soveraign Ladies remembrance in the breasts and loves of those persons of honour and quality, that presented most of these rare Receipts to her. And now that my age will not suffer me, as I fell with the Court, to remain much longer in this troublesome World, I thought it my duty, if I could not do her Majesty further service, at least to use my best endeavours to prevent all disservices that might be done to her. I make no question, though I have thus faithfully vindicated my self, that there are some persons still left, that will view this Volume with a kinde of indignation, that these Copies should be made publique by a Servant, which were onely intrusted to so sacred a Custody; I acknowledge, if they finde any of them altered or corrupted by the failings of printing, I am exposed to their just angers, as some of their names are particularly affixed; but I hope my absence in the Countrey may in part plead for me against those familiar Errata's, which are incident to all Editions; more especially since my infirm age could not permit me with my constant endeavours to attend the Press, insomuch that I must ingenuously confess, some

Re-

The Epistle

Receipts are disordered in their placing, others false Printed; which kinde of dealing I must impute to the more unfortunate customs of Printers, whose trivial excuses cannot free me from the highest misfortune that may befall me on this earth. Should my Royal Mistress be displeased, from the Bar of whose resentments I can make no appeal, but as I hope she may smile at the happy recovery of those Papers, which perhaps these troubles, and her travels, might utterly have deprived her of, had not my diligent care preserved them for her Majesties review, as also for a more general good. Reader, I am sorrowful that I have detained thee so long from thy more beneficial use of this Book; thank the times, not me, for otherwise these precious leaves, had never been in common, I have no more to write, but that I am.

Your truly loving Friend,

W. M.

The Prescribers, and Approvers of most of these rare Receipts, there following names are in several Pages of this Book inserted and annexed to their own experienced Receipts.

King Edward *the sixth*   Page 272
Queen Elizabeth   272
King Charles *the first*   30
Queen Mary   31
Lady Elizabeth *daughter to* King Charles *the first*   256
Dr. Mayhern *Physician to the late* King   180
Dr.

The Approvers Names.

Dr. Bates	186
Dr. King	284
Dr. Mountford	290
Dr. Forster	176, 177
Dr. More	178
Dr. Butler	1, 2, 293
Dr. Bassa *an Italian*	7, 8
Dr. Adrian Gilbert	11
Dr. Atkinson	17, 160
Dr. Goffe	121
Dr. Stephens	21, 87, 140, 275
Dr. Price	24
Dr. Read	39
Dr. May	47
Dr. Blacksmith	55, 56, 83
Dr. Brasdale	59
Dr. Frier	55, 173
Dr. Atkins	65, 73, 74, 83
Dr. Gifford	3
Dr. Twine	82, 288
Dr. Wetherborn	89
Dr. Lewkener	134, 154
Dr. Eglestone	136
Dr. Soper	147
Mr. Stepkins *Occulist*	18, 130
Mr. Fenton *Chyrur.*	24
Mr. Francis Cox *Chyrur.*	66
Mr. Lumley *Chyrur.*	123
Mr Thomas Potter *Chyrur.*	145

Mr.

The Approvers Names.

Mr. Phillips *Apothecary*	296
B. Laud *Arch-Bishop of Canterbury*	275
Bishop of Worcester	19
Earl of Arundel CC.	3
Lord *Treasurer*	32
Lord Bacon *Vic. of St.* Albans	281
Lord Vic. Conway CC.	99
Lord Spencer	283
Lord Sheffeld	62
Sir Walter Raleigh	274
Sir Thomas Mayner	33
Sir Edward Terrel	40
Sir Edward Bolstward	72
Sir Edward Spencer	28
Sir Kenelm Digby	290
Mr. *Justice* Hutton	191
Countess of Arundel	25, 49, 168
Countess of Worcester	69
Countess of Oxford	156
Countess of Kent	274
Countess of Rutland CC.	109
Lady Mounteagle	141
Lady Abergany CC.	42
Lady Nevel	147, 163
Lady Spotswood	286
Lady Drury	44
Lady Gifford	299
Lady Hobby	11
Lady Leonard	158

Lady

The Approvers Names.

Lady Smith	159
Lady Goring	161, 162
Lady Mildmay	164
Lady Bray	167
Lady Dacres	168
Lady Thornborough	267
Lady Mallet	275
Mrs. Duke	114
Mrs. Covet	6
Mrs. Lee C.C.	82
Mrs. Powel	166
Mrs. Jones	164
Mrs Chaunce	165
Mrs. Shelly C.C.	38
Mr. Edward Houghton	166
Mr. Lucarello	170
Mr. Elderton	170
Mr. Rodstone C.C.	51
Mr. Ferene *the Queens Perfumer*	273

THE QUEENS CABINET OPENED:
OR,
The Pearle of Practice.
Accurate, Physical, and Chyrurgical Receipts.

Doctor Butler's Preservative against the Plague.

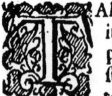Ake Wood sorrel, and pick it from the stalk, and pound it very well in a stone Mortar; then take to every pound of beaten Sorrel a pound of Sugar finely beaten, and two ounces of Mithridate, beat them very well together, and put them in pots for your use; take every morning before

and

and after the infection for some time together of this Conserve, as much as a Walnut.

Dr. Butlers *Cordial Water*.

Take Pimpernel, Carduus, Angelica, Scordium, Scabious, Dragon, and still these severally in a Rose still; and when you have a pint of the water of every of these sorts of Hearbs, then mingle all these together very well, and dissolve in it half a pound of Venice Treacle, then still all these together, and mingle the stronger water with the small, six spoonfuls of this water, made blood warm, given to one sick of the Plague, driveth all venome from the heart. It is excellent, so used, for the Small Pox, or for any pestilent Feaver.

Dr. Butlers *Purging Ale*.

Take of Sarsaparilla two ounces, of Polypody of the Oak, and Sena, of each four ounces, Caroway-seed, and Anifeeds, of each half an ounce, Liquorish two ounces, Maidenhair and Agrimony, of each one little handful; Scurvey half a bushel; beat all these grosly, and put them into a course Canvas bag, and

and hang it into three gallons of strong Ale; when it is three dayes old drink it.

Dr. Giffords *Amber Pills for a Consumption.*

Take of Venice Turpentine one ounce washed, and six graines of the powder of white Amber, mixt them together, and set them in a clean pot upon embers, and let it not stand too hot; to try whether it be enough, take a drop, and let it cool; if after it is cold it be stiffe, and will not cleave to the finger, it is enough: then take of the powders of Pearl, White Amber, and Coral, of each a quantity, as a quarter of an ounce, of the inner bark of an Oak a quarter of an ounce, of Cinamon and Nutmegs of each as much, and three ounces of hard white Sugar; make all these into a powder, and seeth them, and put the pills into them; before you take them, you must be well purged, after which you must take three of the aforesaid Pills wrapped up in the powder, what else you will, and in the morning take the yolk of a new laid Egg warmed a little, and put into it as much of the powder as will lie on a shilling, and

and sup it off; let this be used some time together, and there will be great benefit found by it.

To comfort the Heart and Spirits, and to suppress Melancholly.

Take of the juyces of Borage and Buglosse, of each one pint and a half, juyce of Pippins, or Queen Apples one pint, juyce of Balm half a pint, clarifie them, then take Chochenel made into powder four drams; infuse it in the said juyces being cold in an earthen pan for two dayes, stirring it often, then strain it, and with four pound of powder Sugar, (or two pound if you mean not to keep it long) boyl it to a syrrup, then take it off, and when it is almost cold, put to it Diamargaritum Frigidum one dram and a half, Diambra four scruples. Take thereof a spoonful or two for many mornings together, and when you awake in the night, if there be cause; you may also adde to some part of it Saffron to make it more cordial, by putting some powder of Saffron in a linnen clout tied up, and so milking it out into the syrrup, let the substance there-

thereof remain in the cloth, and take thereof sometimes. *Approved.*

A Cordial Electuary for stuffing of the stomach, or shortness of breath.

Take a pint of the best Honey, set it on the fire and scum it clean, then put to a bundle of hysop bruised small before you tie it up; let it boil well, till the Honey taste of the Hysop, then strain out the Honey very hard, and put to it the powder of Angelica root, the weight of six pence, powder of Elicampane root the weight of six pence, Ginger and Pepper, of each the weight of two pence, Liquorish and Anniseed of each the weight of eight pence, all beaten very small severally: put all these into the strained Honey, and let them boil a little space, stirring them well together all the time, then take them from the fire, and pour all into a clean gallypot, stirring it alwayes till it be through cold, and keep it close covered for your use. When any are troubled with stuffing at the Stomach, or shortness of breath, let them take of this Electuary with a bruised Liquorish stick, and they shall

shall sensibly finde much good by it. This was Queen *Elizabeths* Electuary for these infirmities.

Mr. Covets Medicine for the Palsie.

Take a pint of the strongest mustard, set it in an Oven for two or three times, till it be as thick as a hasty pudding, the Oven must not be too hot to burn it; then set it on a chafing-dish of coals, till it be dry enough to make into powder. Take half an ounce of Betony powder, and mix it with the said powder, and sweeten it with Sugar-candy to your taste. Take of this every morning for ten dayes. *Approved.*

A Receipt to help Digestion.

Take two quarts of small Ale, put to it red mints one handful, as much of red Sage, a little Cinnamon; let it boyl softly till half be wasted; sweeten it with Sugar to your taste, and drink thereof a draught morning and evening.

A singular Cordial.

Take two ounces of dried red Gillyflowers, and put them into a pottle of Sack, put to it three ounces of fine Sugar in powder, and half a scruple of Ambergreese in powder; put all these in a stone bottle, stop it close with a strong cork, and shake it oft After it hath stood ten dayes, pass it through a Jelly bagg, and give two or three spoonfuls of it for a great Cordial. This way you may also make Lavander wine for the Palsie, and other diseases.

Dr. Bassa an Italian. An approved Receipt to break the Stone in the Kidneys.

In the moneth of *May* distill Cowdung, then take two live Hares, and strangle them in their blood, then take the one of them, and put it into an earthen vessel or pot, and cover it well with a mortar made of horse dung and hay, and bake it in an Oven with houshold bread, and let it still in an Oven two or three dayes, baking a new with any thing, untill the Hare be baked or dried to powder; then beat it well, and keep it for your use. The other Hare you must flea, and take out the guts onely, then distill all the rest, and keep this water: then take at the new and full of the Moon, or any other time, three mornings together as much of this powder as will lie on six pence, with two spoonfuls of each water; and it will break any stone in the Kidneys.

Dr. Basse. Remedy for a bloody Urine, or to break a Stone in the Bladder.

Take the distilled water of Saxifrage, Coriander, Parsley, and cod of broom when they be green, the berries of white Thorn, stilled when they be ripe; they must be stamped stones and all, and then distilled: the green hulls of Walnuts when they be ripe stilled, Raysins of the sun stilled; every one of these waters must be stilled by it self. Then take an equal quantity of each, as a pint of *Aqua Spirita*; put them all together, and still them in an ordinary still, or in *B.* after scum the water nine or ten dayes: and take of this water for ten or fifteen dayes, five or six spoonfuls

fuls a time in the morning fasting, and use to take it after a day or two once in a moneth.

Syrup of Turnips.

First bake the Turnips in a pot with houshold bread, then press out the Liquor between two platters; put a pint of this liquour to half a pint of Hysop water, and as much brown Sugarcandy as will sweeten it; and boil it to the consistence of a Syrup. It is very good for a Cold or Consumption.

Syrup of Citron Peels.

Take the outermost fresh Peels of Citrons cut in small pieces, and pour on them two quarts of water, then wring it through a cloth; put to the liquour one pound of powder sugar, boil it to a Syrup, and when it is sodden, put four grains of Musk to it, dissolved in Damask Rose water. This Syrup cooleth not. It defendeth from the Plague.

A Cordial Syrup to cleanse the blood, open Obstructions, prevent a Consumption, &c.

Take Rosemary flowers, Betony, Clove-gilly-flowers, Borrage, Broom, Cowslip flowers, Red-rose-leaves, Melilot, Comfrey, Clarey, Pimpinel flowers, of each two ounces, red Currans four pounds: infuse all these into six quarts of Claret Wine, put to it fourteen pounds of ripe Elder berries, make the Wine scalding hot, then put in the Flowers, Currans, and Elder berries, cover the pot, and paste it very close, set it in a kettle of warm water to infuse fourty eight hours, till the vertue of the ingredients be all drawn out, then press it out hard, and put to every pint of the liquour one pound and three quarters of powder Sugar, boil and scum it, till you finde the Syrup thick enough, when it is cold bottle it, and keep it for your use. Take two spoonfuls in a morning, and so much in the afternoon, fasting two hours after it.

A Medicine for a Dropsie, approved by the Lady Hobby, *who was cured her self by it.*

Take Carowayes, Smallage, Time, Hysop, Water-cresses, Penniroyal, Nettle tops, Calamint, Elecampane-roots, of each one little handful, Horse radish two pounds, boil them in six quarts of running water, until half be consumed, then strain it, boil it a new with a pottle of Canary Sack, Liquorish twelve ounces, sweet Fennel-seed, one ounce bruised, and a quarter of an ounce of Cumin-seed bruised; boil all these above half an hour, then strain it, and keep it for your use; nine spoonfuls in the morning fasting, and as much at three or four a clock in the afternoon, use it for some time together. This the Lady *Hobby* proved by her self.

Dr. Adrian Gilberts *most soveraign cordial Water.*

Take Spearmint, Broom-mint, Mother of Time, the Blossome tops of Garden Time, red Penniroyal, Scabious, Celandine, Wood Sorrel, Wood Betony, An-

Angelica leaves and stalkes, set Wall leaves, Peony leaves, Egrimony, Tormentil, sweet Marjoram, red Sage, Rue, Rossolis, Angelica roots, Elecampany roots, set Wall roots, green Peniroyal, Comfrey blossoms and leaves, Juniper berries, of each a pound, Balm, Carduus, Benedictus, Dragon, Feaverfew, Wormwood, of each two pounds; steep all these in the Lees of strong pure venient Claret Wine for nine dayes, every day twice turning them to mingle them well in the Lees, then distill them in a Limbeck with a red clear head, with two pounds of shaved Harts-horn, and Ivory twelve ounces; draw as long of it as you may in several pottle glasses: the first is accounted the best and uncompounded, and the perfectest against the Plague, spotted Feavers, small Pocks, ordinary Feavers, divers times experienced by my self, either to prevent, or in the time of these sicknesses. If you will compound it because the water hath an ill taste, then take the first gallon of the water, and mix it with a pottle of the best Malaga sack, and put into them three pounds of Raisins *solis* stoned, Figs one pound and a half, the flowers of Clove-gilly-flowers,

ers, Cowslips and Marigolds, blue Violets, of each two pounds, red Rose buds one pound, Ambergreese, Bezoar stone, clarified Sugar, Aniseeds, Liquorish, and what else you please.

These are *Adrian Gilberts* Receipts, having had experience of them most constantly sure. The uncompounded water is the more excellent: and if in time of infection one take two spoonfuls of it in good Beer or white Wine, he may safely walk from danger by the leave of God. If any of the former diseases attach any person, then he must take four ounces of the first water, and mix therewith either the Syrups of Violets, Clove-gilly-flowers, or Angelica, as the disease is; one spoonful of the Syrup is sufficient for four ounces of the water, so take it in three times.

For a swoln Face.

Take Oyl of Elder and Plantain-water, of each one ounce, beat them well together, until they be exactly incorporated, and therewith anoint the tumefied place twice or thrice in a day, until the swelling be chased away.

Cock

Cock water for a Consumption.

Take a running Cock, pull him alive, then kill him, cut him abroad by the back, take out the entrails, and wipe him clean, then quarter him, and break his bones; then put him into a Rose water still, with a pottle of sack, Currans, and Raisins solis stoned, and Figs sliced, of each one pound, Dates stoned and cut small half a pound, Rosemary flowers, Wilde Time, Spearmint, of each one handful, Organs or Wilde Marjoram, Bugloss, Pimpinel, of each two handfuls, and a bottle of new milk from a red cow. Distill these with a soft fire, put into the Receiver a quarter of a pound of brown Sugarcandy beaten small, four grains of Ambergreese, fourty grains of prepared Pearl, and half a book of leaf Gold cut very small; you must mingle the strong water with the small, and let the Patient take two spoonfuls of it in the morning, and as much at going to bed.

A precious Cordial for a sick body.

Take three spoonfuls of Mint water, and

and as much of Muscadine and Wormwood water, two or three spoonfuls of fine Sugar, and two or three drops of Cinnamon spirit; beat these well together with two or three spoonfuls of Clove-gilly-flowers spirit, and give the Patient now and then one spoonfull thereof, especially when he or she goeth to bed.

Wormwood Cakes good for a cold Stomach, and to help Digestion.

Take pube searced Sugar two ounces, and wet it with the Spirit of Wormwood, then take a little Gum Tragiganth, and steep it all night in Rose water, then take some of this and the wet Sugar, and beat them together in an Alablaster Mortar, till it come to a paste like dough, if you please put a little Musk to it, then make it up in little cakes of the breadth of a groat or three pence; lay them upon plates, and dry them gently in an Oven, and keep them in a dry place for your use: and upon occasion hold one of them in your mouth to melt, and swallow the dissolved juyce thereof for the infirmities aforesaid.

To make water of Life.

Take Balm leaves and stalks, Burnet leaves and flowers, Rosemary, red Sage, Taragon, Tormentil leaves, Rossolis, red Roses, Carnation, Hysop, Thyme, red strings that grow upon Savory, red Fennel leaves and roots, red Mints, of each one handful; bruise these hearbs and put them in a great earthen pot, and pour on them as much white Wine as will cover them, stop them close, and let them steep for eight or nine dayes, then put to it Cinnamon, Ginger, Angelica seeds, Cloves and Nutmegs, of each one ounce, a little Saffron, Sugar one pound, Raysins *Solis* stoned one pound, Dates stoned and sliced half a pound, the loines and legs of an old Coney, fleshy running Capon, the red flesh of the sinnews of a leg of Mutton, four young Chickens, twelve Larks, the yolks of twelve Eggs, a Loaf of white bread cut in sops, and two or three ounces of Mithridate or Treacle, and as much Bastard, or Muscadine as will cover them all. Distill all with a moderate fire, and keep the first and second waters by themselves,

selves; and when there comes no more by distilling, put more Wine into the Pot upon the same stuff, and distill it again, and you shall have another good water. This water must be kept in a double glass close stopt very carefully: it is good against many infirmities, as the Dropsie, Palsie, Ague, Sweating, Spleen, Worms, Yellow and Black Jaundies; it strengthneth the Spirits, Brain, Heart, Liver, and Stomach. Take two or three spoonfuls when need is by it self: or with Ale, Beer, or wine mingled with Sugar.

Dr. Atkinsons *excellent Perfume against the Plague*.

Take Angelica roots, and dry them a very little in an Oven, or by the fire; and then bruise them very soft, and lay them in Wine Vinegar to steep, being close covered three or four days, and then heat a brick hot, and lay the same thereon every morning; this is excellent to air the house or any clothes, or to breath over in the morning fasting.

To make Saffron water.

Take seven Quarts of white Wine, and infuse in it all night one ounce of Saffron dryed, and in the morning distill it in a Limbeck, or Glass body with a head, and put some white Sugar-candy finely beaten into the Receiver for it to drop on.

Mr. Stepkins Water for the Eyes.

Take four ounces of white Rose water, and two drams of Tutia in powder, shake them well together in a glass vial, and drop of it a little into the Eyes evening and morning, it is very good for any hot Rheum.

A precious Water to revive the Spirits.

Take four gallons of strong Ale, five ounces of Aniseeds, Liquorish scraped half a pound, sweet Mints, Angelica, Betony, Cowslip flowers, Sage and Rosemary flowers, sweet Marjoram, of each three handfuls, Pelitory of the wall one handful. After it is for two or three dayes,

dayes, distill it in a Limbeck, and in the water infuse one handful of the flowers aforesaid, Cinnamon and Fennel-seed of each half an ounce, Juniper berries bruised one dram, Red-rose buds, roasted Apples, and Dates sliced and stoned, of each half a pound, distill it again, and sweeten it with some Sugar-candy, and take of Ambergreese, Pearle, red Coral, Harts-horn powdred, and leaf Gold, of each half a dram; put them into a fine linnen bag, and hang it by a thread in a glass.

The Bishop of Worcesters admirably curing Powder.

Take black tips of Crabs claws when the Sun enters into *Cancer*, which is every year on the eleventh day of *June*; pick and wash them clean, and beat them into fine powder, which finely searce, then take Musk and Civet, of each three grains, Ambergreese twelve grains, rub them in the bottom of the Mortar, and then beat them and the powdar of the Claws together; then with a pound of this powder mix one ounce of the magistery of Pearle. Then take ten skins of
Adders,

Adders or Snakes, or Slow worm, cut them in pieces, and put them into a pipkin to a pint and a half of Spring water, cover it close, and set it on a gentle fire to simmer onely, not to boil, for ten or twelve hours, in which time it will be turned into a Jelly, and therewith make the said powder into balls. If such skins are not to be gotten, then take six ounces of shaved Harts-horn, and boil it to a Jelly, and therewith make the said powder into balls; the horn must be of a red Deer kil'd in *August*, when the moon is in *Leo*, for that is best. The Dose is seven or eight grains in beer or wine.

To make Spirit of Castoreum.

Take Calamints four ounces, Orange peels two ounces, Nep half a handful, Walnut blossoms half an ounce, Rosemary flowers, and tops of Sage, of each one handful, Castoreum one ounce, white Wine one quart; distill them in a Limbeck. This Water is good for swounding fits, weak stomachs, and rising of the Mother.

A Water for the Stone.

Take a quart of clean pickt Strawberries, put them in a glass, pour on them a quart of Aqua vitæ, let them stand and steep; and take two or three spoonfuls of it morning and evening with fine Sugar, or white Sugarcandy. It will keep all the year. *Approved.*

To make Dr. Stephens Water.

Take a gallon of Claret wine or Sack, Cinnamon, Ginger, Grains of Paradise, Gallingall, Nutmegs, Aniseed, and Fennel-seed, of each three drams, Sage, Mint, red Roses, Pellitory of the Wall, Wilde Marjoram, Rosemary, Wilde Time, Cammomil, Lavender, of each one handful: bruise the said spices small, cut and bruise the Hearbs, and put all into the Wine in a Limbeck, and after it hath stood twenty four hours, distill it gently, and keep the first water by it self, and so the second.

For a Tetter.

Take water of red Tar, and wash it therewith. This is an approved remedy.

A special water for a Consumption.

Take a peck of garden shell Snails, wash them in small Beer, put them into a great Iron dripping-pan, and set them on the hot fire of Charcoals, and keep them constantly stirring till they make no noise at all; then with a knife and cloth pick them out, and wipe them clean, then bruise them in a stone Mortar, shells and all; then take a quart of Earth Worms, rip them up with a knife, and scoure them with Salt, and wash them clean, and beat them in the Mortar; then take a large clean Brass pot to distill them in, put into it two handfuls of Angelica, on them lay two handfuls of Celandine, a quart of Rosemary flowers, of Betony and Agrimony, of each two handfuls; Bears-foot, Red dock leaves, the bark of Barberies, and Wood Sorrel, of each one handful, Rice half a handful, Funugreek and Turnerick, of each

each one ounce, Saffron dryed and beaten into powder the weight of six pence, Harts-horn and Cloves beaten, of each three ounces; when all these are in the Pot, put the Snails and Worms upon them, and then pour on them three gallons of strong Ale; then set on the Limbeck, and paste it close with Rye dough, that no air come out or get in, and so let it stand one and twenty hours, and distill it with a moderate fire, and receive the several Quarts in several Glasses close stopt. The Patient must take every morning fasting, and not sleep after it, two spoonfuls of the strongest water, and four spoonfuls of the weakest at one time, fasting two hours after it.

Syrup of Pearmains good against Melancholy.

Take one pound of the juyce of Pearmains, boil it with a soft fire till half be consumed; then put it in a glass, and there let it stand till it be setled; and put to it as much of the juyce of the leaves and roots of Borage, Sugar half a pound, syrup of Citrons three ounces; let them boil together to the consistence of a syrup

Tincture

Tincture of Ambergreese.

Put into half a pint of pure spirit of Wine in a strong glass, Ambergreese one ounce, Musk two drams, stop the glass close with a cork and bladder, and set it in hot horse dung twelve dayes; then pour off the Spirit gently, and put as much new spirit on, and do as before, and pour it off clean: after all this the Ambergreese will serve for ordinary uses. One drop of this Tincture will perfume any thing; besides it is a great Cordial.

Dr. Price, *and Mr.* Fenton *the Chyrurgion, their excellent Medicine for the Plague after Infection.*

Take assoon as you find your self sick, as much Diascordium as the weight of a shilling, with ten grains of the powder called *Speciei de gemmis*, well mingled together; and streight after this let the party drink a good draught of hot posset ale made with Carduus Benedictus, Sorrel, Scabiosa, and Scordium, within eight hours after the first taking of it, the

the party must take the Diascordium, and Posset again as aforesaid, and in like sort the third time within eight hours after, but not above three times, nor the third time, if the party mend, after the first or second taking. Doctor *Price* doth commend much thereof to be taken for the kinde of cure for the Plague after one is infected; and Mr. *Frenton* the excellent Chyrurgeon, who hath much experience in the cure of the Plague, doth highly commend it as a thing in his own experience proved very good. The use of a root called Sedour is to be chewed in the mouth, still when one is in the company of such persons as are thought to be infected with the contagition: this root is to be bought at the Apothecaries.

A drink for the Plague or pestilent Feaver proved by the Countess of Arundel, in the year 1603.

Take a pint of Malmsey and burn it, and put thereto a spoonful of grains, being bruised, and take four spoonfuls of the same in a porringer, and put therein a spoonful of Jean Treacle, and give

give the Patient to drink as hot as he can suffer it, and let him drink a draught of the Malmsey after it, and so sweat: if he be vehemently infected, he will bring the Medicine up again; but you must apply the same very often day and night till he brook it; for so long as he doth bring it up again, there is danger in him: but if he once brook it, there is no doubt of his recovery by the Grace of God: provided then when the party infected hath taken the aforesaid Medicine and sweateth, if he bring it up again, then you must give him the aforesaid quantity of Malmsey and grains, but no Treacle, for it will be too hot for him, being in a sweat. This Medicine is proved, and the party hath recovered, and the sheets have been found full of blue marks, and no sore hath come forth; this being taken in the beginning of the sickness. Also this Medicine saved 38 Commons of *Windsor* the last great Plauge 1593 was proved upon many poor people, and they recovered.

A

A Syrup for a Cold.

Take Penniroyal half an ounce, Raisins of the Sun stoned one ounce, half so much Liquorish bruised, boil them in a pint of running water, till half be consumed; then strain it out hard, and with Sugar boil it to a pretty thick Syrup, and take it with a Liquorish stick: *Often proved.*

An excellent Receipt for a precious water.

Take a pottle of the second water of Aqua Composita, of Balm, Betony, Pellitory of the Wall, sweet Marjoram, the flowers of Cowslip, Rosemary, and Sage, of each one handful, the seeds of Anise, Caroway, Coriander, Fennil, and Gromel, and Juniper berries, of each one spoonful, three or four Nutmegs, Cinnamon one ounce, two or three large Mace; bruise all these, and let them lye ten dayes in steep in the Aqua Composita; set the glass in the Sun, and stir it well every morning, then strain it, and put to it three quarters of a pound of fine Sugar, one graine of Ambergreese, and two graines of Musk.

To make an excellent Syrup of Citrons, or Lemons without fire.

Take Citrons, or Limons, as many as you will, pare off their rindes, then slice them very thin; then put into silver, or glass bason, a thick lay of fine Sugar, and upon that the slices of Citrons or Lemons, and lay after lay of Sugar, and the other, till the bason be near full; let it stand all night covered with a paper, the next day pour of the Liquor into a glass through a Tiffany strainer; be sure you put sugar enough to them at the first, and it will keep a whole year good, if it be set well up.

A Salve for the Eyes, made by Sir Edward Spencer.

Take new Hogs greese tried and clarified two ounces, steep it six hours in Red-rose-water; after wash it in the best White Wine, wherein Lapis Calaminaris hath been twelve times quenched: it will take a pottle of White Wine, for the

the Lapis Calaminaris will waste it by often quenching, a piece of the Lapis as big as a Turkey Egg will serve; when the grease is well washed, adde to it one ounce of Lapis Tutia prepared, of Lapis Hematites well washed, two scruples, Aloes Succotrina twelve grains, Pearle four grains; all these must be prepared and made into fine powder, put to it some red Fennel-water, and make it into a Salve. If the eyes be very ill, put into each corner of them as much as a pins head of this Salve; and if the eyes be exceeding sore, anoint therewith onely the Eye-lids. As the Salve drieth, put to it red Fennel water to keep it moist.

For the Small Pocks or Measles.

Take an ounce of Treacle, half an ounce of set Wall cut small, a penniworth of Saffron ground small; mix them, and take thereof in a morning upon a knives point as much as you can take up at twice or thrice three mornings together.

A very good Glyster for the winde.

Take Mallow leaves, Cammomill, Mercury, Pelitory of the Wall, Mugwort and Penniroyal, of each a small handful, Melilot and Cammomil flowers, of each half a handful, of the seeds of Anise, Caroway, Cummin and Fennel, of each one quarter of an ounce; Bayberries and Juniper berries, of each three drams; boil all these in three pints of clear posset ale to twelve ounces, and use it warm.

The Kings Medicine for the Plague.

Take a little handful of Hearb-grace, as much of Sage, the like quantity of Elder leaves, as much of Red Bramble leaves, stamp them altogether, and strain them through a fair linnen cloth, with a quart of White wine, and a quantity of white Vinegar, and a quantity of white Ginger, and mingle all together; after the first day you shall be safe four and twenty dayes: after the ninth day a whole year by the grace of God; and if it fortune that one be strucken with the

the Plague before he hath drunk the Medicine, then take the aforesaid with a spoonful of Scabiosa, and a spoonful of Betony water, and a quantity of fine Treacle, and put them together, and cause the Patient to drink it, and it will put out all venome; and if it fortune that the botch appear, take the leaves of red Brambles, Elder leaves, and Mustard seed, stamp them together, and make a plaister thereof, and lay it to the sore, and it will draw out all the venome, and the person shall be whole by the Grace of God.

A Medicine for the Plague that the Lord Mayor had from the Queen.

Take of Sage, Elder, and red Bramble leaves, of each one little handful; stamp and strain them together through a cloth with a quart of White Wine, then take a quantity of White Vinegar, and mingle all these together, and drink thereof morning and night a spoonful at a time nine dayes together, and you shall be whole. There is no Medicine more excellent then this, when the sore doth appear, then to take a cock Chick and Pullet; and let the rump be bare, and hold the rump of the said Chick to the sore, and it will gape and labour for life, and in the end dye; then take another, and the third, and so long as any do dye: for when the poyson is quite drawn out, the Chick will live, the sore presently will asswage, and the party recover. Mr. *Winlour* proved this upon one of his own children; the thirteenth Chick dyed, the fourteenth lived, and the party cured.

Lord Treasurers Receipt for an Ague.

Take a quantity of Plantain, shred it, and double distill it, and take six or eight sponfuls of the water, with as much Borage-water, with a little Sugar, and one Nutmeg; and drink it warm in the cold fit, by Gods help it will cure you.

For Rhume in the Eyes.

Take one spoonful of Commin-seed finely beaten, and boil it in Verjuyce till half be consumed; put to it it some course wheat bran, and boil it till it be dry, then put it in a small linnen bag, and lay it to the nape of the neck so hot as you can endure it, and it will draw the Rhume away.

To break the Stone, and bring away the Gravel.

Take the inner bark of a red Filberd-tree, and shave a good handful of it, and take as much Saxifrage, and steep them in a quart of Ale or white Wine, and drink a good draught thereof nine mornings together fasting.

A Cordial Water in the time of Infection, by Sir Thomas Mayner.

Take the juyce of green Walnut shells and all two pound, the juyces of Balm, Carduus Benedictus, and Marigolds, of each three pounds, roots of great Docks half a pound, Butchers broom roots, and all three quarters of a pound, Angelica and Masterwort of each three ounces, Scordium leaves two handfuls, Treacle Venice and Mithridate of each four ounces, Canary Wine three pints, juyce of Limons one pint, digest these in a glass body two dayes close stopt, then put on a glass head, and distill it, and when it is half distilled, strain that which is left in the glasse through a linnen cloth, and distill it till it grow thick as Honey, which put into a Gally-pot, and give some of it in the time of Infection on a knifes point. The distilled water is also good for the same purpose.

China broth for a Consumption.

Take one ounce of China root chipped thin, and steep it in three pints of water all night on embers covered, the next day take a Cock chicken deplumed and exenterated, and put in its belly Agrimony, Maidenhair, of each half a handful, Raisins of the Sun stoned one good handful, and as much French barley; boil all these in a pipkin close covered on a gentle fire for six or seven hours, let it stand till it be cold, strain it, or let it run through a Hypocras bag, and keep it in a glasse for your use. Take a good draught of it in the morning, and at four a clock in the afternoon.

A comfortable bag for the Stomach.

Take Balm, Wormwood, Rosemary, Spearmints, Sweet Marjoram, Winter savory, of each half a handful, dry them between two dishes on a chafing-dish of coals, sprinkling them often with good Vinegar; when they are well dryed, put to them some crumbs of bread, Cloves, Cinnamon, and Nutmeg beaten to powder; put them in a fine linnen bag, quilt it, and lay it warm to the Stomach.

To encrease Womans milk.

Bruise Fennel seed, and boil them in Barley water, and let the Woman drink thereof often.

To expel Winde.

Take a handful of Groundswel stripped downwards, as much of Sage, and a quarter of a pound of Currans, boil these in a pint of Ale, and drink it.

For the Piles.

Take white Lead finely scraped one dram, burnt Allum two drams temper them with Hogs Lard and Plantan-water, and therewith anoint the grieved place.

For a Thrush, or Canker in the Mouth.

Take two spoonfuls of clarified Honey, and put a piece of Allum between red hot tongs, and hold it till it drop into the Honey, and therewith dress the mouth often, until it be perfectly cured.

A green Oyntment good for Bruises, Swellings, and Wrenches in Man, Horse, or other Beast.

Take six pound of *May* Butter unsalted, Oyl-Olive one quart, Barrows-grease four pound, Rosin and Turpentine of each one pound, Frankincense half a pound; then take these following Hearbs of each one handful: Balm, Smallage, Lovage, Red Sage, Lavander, Cotten, Marjoram, Rosemary, Mallows, Camomil, Plaintain, Alheal, Chick-

Chickweed, Rue, Parsley, Comfrey, Laurel leaves, Birch leaves, Longwort, English Tobacco, Groundswel, Woundwort, Agrimony, Briony, Carduus Benedictus, Betony, Adders Tongue, Saint Johns-wort, pick all these, wash them clean, and strain the water clean from them. These hearbs must be gathered after Sun rising. Stamp them very small in a stone Mortar, then beat the Rosin and Frankincense to powder, and melt them alone; then put in the Oyl, Butter, and Hogs greafe, and when all is well melted, put in the Hearbs, and let them boil half a quarter of an hour, then take it from the fire, and scum it very clean a quarter of an hour; and when it is off the fire, put in the Turpentine, and two ounces of Verdigreese, stir it well, or else it will run over, and so stir it till it leave boiling; then put it in an earthen pot, which stop very close with a cloath, and a board on the top, and set it in a Horse Dunghill 21 dayes; and take it out, and put it into a Kettle, and let it boil a little, taking heed that it boil not over, then strain it through a course cloth, and put to it half a pound of Oyl of Spike,

Spike, and cover the pot close till you use it. When you have any occasion to use it, warm it a little for a cold cause, and anoint the place grieved. Mix this Oyl with the like quantity of the Oyl of Bayes, when it is for a Melander in a Horse, or a dry itch in a Horse or Mare; then take Quick-silver, and beat it often with fasting spittle, till it be killed and look black, and take a quart of Comfrey to the quantity of Quick-silver, to which put thrice so much of the said Oyl; beat all well together, and use it. For a man it must be well chafed in the Palme of the hand three or four times. If you use it for a Horse, put to it Brimstone finely beaten, and work it altogether, as aforesaid.

An excellent Sear-cloth for a Wound, Bruise, or Ach.

Take a pint of Oyl Olive, four ounces of Unguentum Populeon, the Oyls of Cammomel and Roses, of each one ounce, Virgins Wax three ounces, Red lead in powder eight ounces; boil these together, continually stirring them, till they will stick to a cloth, which

which is enough, then wet your clothes in them, and hang them up to dry. The best time to make it is in *March*.

Dr. Reads *Perfume to smell against the Plague*.

First take half a pint of red Rose water, and put thereto the quantity of a hazle Nut of Venice Treacle or Mithridate, stirring them together till they be well infused, then put thereto a quarter of an ounce of Cinnamon broken into small pieces, and bruised in a Mortar, twelve Cloves bruised, the quantity of an hazle Nut of Angelica root sliced very thin, as much of Setwal roots sliced, three or four spoonfuls of White Wine Vinegar; so put them altogether in a glasse, and stop it very close, and shake it two or three times a day together, so keep it to your use, when you wet the spunge, shake the glass: in the Winter you may put to it three or four spoonfuls of Cinnamon water or Sack.

A Perfume against the Plague.

Divers good Physicians opinions are, that to burn Tar every morning in a chafing-dish of coals is most excellent against the Plague; also put in a little Wine Vinegar to the Tar. It is most excellent and approved.

Sir Edward Tertils *Salve, called the chief of all Salves.*

Take Rosin eight ounces, Virgins Wax and Frankincense, of each four ounces, Mastick one ounce, Harts Suet four ounces, Camphire two drams; beat the Rosin, Mastick, and Frankincense in a Mortar together to fine powder; then melt the Rosin and Wax together, then put in the powders: and when they are well melted, strain it through a cloth into a pottle of White Wine, and boil it together, till it be somewhat thick; then let it cool, and put in the Camphire and four ounces of Venice Turpentine drop by drop, lest it clumper, stirring it continually; then make it up into Rolls, and do with it to the

the pleasure of God, and health of man.

The Vertues and use of it.

1. It is good for all wounds and sores, old or new, in any place.
2. It cleanseth all Festers in the flesh, and heals more in nine dayes, then other salves cure in a moneth.
3. It suffers no dead flesh to ingender or abide where it comes.
4. It cureth the head-ache, rubbing the Temples therewith.
5. It cureth a salt fleam face.
6. It helpeth Sinews that grow stiff, or spring with labor, or wax dry for want of blood.
7. It draweth out rusty Iron, Arrow-heads, Stubs, Splints, Thorns, or whatsoever is fixed in the flesh or wound.
8. It cureth the biting of a mad Dog, or pricking of any venemous creature.
9. It cureth all Felons, or white flaws.
10. It is good for all Festering Cankers.
11. It helpeth all Aches of the Liver, Spleen, Kidneys, Back, Sides, Arms, or Legs.
12. It cureth Biles, Blanes, Botches,

Im-

Impostumes, Swellings, and Tumors in any part of the body.

13. It helpeth all aches and pains of the genitors in man or woman.

14. It cureth Scabs, Itch, Wrenches, Sprains, Strains, Gouts, Palsies, Dropsies, and waters between the flesh and skin.

15. It healeth the Hemorrhoides, or Piles in man or woman.

16. It cureth the bloody Flux, if the belly be anointed therewith.

17. Make a Sear-cloth thereof to heal all the above said Maladies, with very many other, which for brevity sake are omitted.

A restorative Broth.

Take a young Cock or Capon, flea it, and cut it in four quarters, take out the bones, and chop the flesh somewhat small, put it into an earthen pot of three quarts with a close cover, and pour on it a quart of good red wine, and a pint of red Rose water, and put to one handful of Currans, ten Dates stoned and cut small, of Rosemary flowers or leaves, and Borage, of each half a handful, then close

close on the cover of the pot very fast, and set the said pot in a big brass pot of water, and let it boil five or six hours, taking heed that the water in the brass pot get not into the other pot: when it is well boiled, let it cool leasurely in the brass pot, and then bruise all with a ladle, and strain out the liquor, whereof take morning and evening four or five spoonfuls blood warm.

For the Piles.

Take one spoonful of white dogs turd, as much white Frankincense, and twenty four grains of Aloes, beat them fine and searce them, then take one spoonful of honey, the yolk of an egg, and as much oyl of Roses, as will make it to an ointment; mingle them well together, and anoint the grieved place; if the sore be inward, wet a Tent of lint in the Oyntment, and put it into the Fundament, and spread some of the ointments on a cloth, and put that on it. This is a present remedy.

For a Sore Throat.

Mingle burnt Alum, the yolk of an Egg, powder of white Dogs-turd, and some Honey together; tye a clout on the end of a stick wet in this mixture, and therewith rub the throat: or mix white Dogs-turd and Honey, spread it on sheeps leather, and apply it to the Throat.

To void Phlegm from the Head, Lungs, or Stomach.

Mix Pelitory roots and Mustard together, and hold it in the mouth, and it will draw out much Phlegm from the Head; but if you boil Pelitory roots, Hysop and Mustard in Wine and Vinegar, and gargle the Throat with it, it will cleanse the Lungs and Stomach perfectly.

The Lady Drury's *Medicine for the Cholick. Proved*

Take a turfe of green Grass, and lay it to the Navil, and let it lie till you

you finde ease, the green side must be laid next to the belly.

A Medicine for one thick of Hearing. Proved.

Take the Garden Dasie-roots, and make juyce thereof, and lay the worst side of the head low upon the bolster, and drop three or four drops thereof into the better Ear, this do three or four days together.

An excellent drink for the Stone.

Take Sussafras and Sussaparilla, of each two ounces shayed small, China-root and Tormentil roots, of each one ounce sliced small, Liquourish half a pound beaten, Anniseed four ounces bruised, steep all these in three gallons of running water for twelve hours, then put to them these Simples following, picked and washed, *viz.* Columbine, Lady mantle, Marsh, Mallow and Moul-ear-roots slit, Hearb Robert, Ribwort, Sanible, Scabious, Agrimony, Colts-foot and Betony, of each two handfuls; boil all these together on a soft fire, till one gallon be consumed, then strain it it out, and keep the liquor in a glass close stopped, then take all what remains in the strainer; put it into the pot again, and pour thereon two gallons of running water, and boil them till half the Liquor be consumed, then strain it out, and put both liquors together, set them on the fire, and put a quart of White Wine to it, and let it boil a while gently and scum it clean, then take it off the fire, and put to it half an ounce of Rhubarb slit, and two ounces of good Sena leaves, and stir them well together, and cover the pot close to keep in the heat, and let it stand all night, and in the morning stir it well, and cover it again, and so let it stand four dayes. Take of this Liquor in the morning fasting, four a clock in the afternoon, and after supper at bed time, at each time the quantity of six ounces, and so used it must be till you feel ease.

To preserve a Woman with Childe from miscarrying.

Put a few Cloves and Cinnamon, with a sprig of Baulm and Rosemary into a pint of Claret Wine, and burn it it altogether, then beat the yolks of six new laid Eggs, and put them into the Wine on the fire, then take the Cock-treading of twelve Eggs, and the white of one Egg, and beat them to an Oyl, take off the white froth from it, and put this Oyl into the Wine, and brew all well together with as much powder Sugar, as will make it of an indifferent sweetness: whereof let the said woman take four spoonfuls at a time, when she feeleth any pain to begin in her back or belly.

To make Childrens Teeth come without pain. Proved.

Take the head of a Hare boiled or roasted, and with the brains thereof mingle Honey and Butter, and therewith anoint the childes gums as often as you please.

Dr. Mays Juice of Liquorish to stay Rhume, and preserve the Lungs.

Take six little handfuls of the tops of Hysop, Rosemary flowers, one little handful, of the leaves of Coltsfoot, four little handfuls, stamp and take the juyce

juyce of them, and put to it a pint of Hyſop-water, or running water; unto all theſe put four ounces of Liquoriſh finely beaten and ſearſed, then ſet it on the fire, and boil it till it be as thick as cream, then ſtrain it through a fine ſtrainer, and ſet it again to the fire, and ſtir it continually till it boil, and put into it boiling four ounces of Yellow Sugar-candy; ſet it boil till it riſe from the bottom, which ſtirring, and when you may handle it, make it up in cakes and rolls as you pleaſe.

To kill a Felon quickly.

Take a little Rue and Sage, ſtamp them ſmall, put to it Oyl of the white of an Egg, and a little Honey, and lay it to the ſore.

A remedy for the pain in the Stomach.

Take a pottle of white Wine, eight ounces of Currans, and four ounces of Elicampane-roots ſliced, a ſprig of Marjoram and Spearmint; boil all theſe together, till the Currans be ſoft, adding to it one ſpoonful of ſweet Fennel ſeed

seed bruised. Drink of the liquor every morning fasting, at four a clock in the afternoon, and when you go to bed the quantity of six spoonfuls. While you drink this, apply to your Stomach one spoonful of Conserve of Roses, two penniworth of Mithridate, Cinnamon, Cloves, and Nutmegs, of each one spoonful, and a penniworth of Saffron, mix these together with Rose-water and Wine Vinegar, and put them in a linnen bag, and warm it, and lay it to the Stomach.

To cure Diseases without taking any thing at the Mouth.

Take one pound of Aloes Hepatica, Myrrhe four ounces, both beaten very fine, *Aqua vitæ* and Rose-water, of each one pint; after one night's infusion distill them in Sand twenty four hours very softly, and in the end make a great fire, and there will come a Balsome, wherewith if you rub the Stomach with a warm cloth dipped therein, it will purge Phlegm and Choler, and all Worms which infect the brain, and breed the Falling-sickness, it expelleth corruptions

ruptions of the Stomach, it helps digestion and appetite, it expurgeth all dross in the bottom of the Stomach, it cureth the Gout being mixed and well beaten with *Aqua vitæ*, and applied warm to the Gouty place, and left long on it.

To break the Stone.

Take Cammock roots, dry them in an Oven, beat them to powder, searse it, and put as much thereof as will lie on a groat into half a pint of white Wine, half a sliced Lemon, a top or two of Rosemary, and some Sugar, let them lie in steep all night, in the morning stir them well together, and drink it off, and wash thereupon a good while. Use this three or four mornings together, and it will make the Stone break, and void away in gravel: but if the Kidneys be ulcerated, then use the Medicine following, *viz.*

To help Ulceration in the Kidneys.

Take two drams of China-root sliced small, Golden rod, Maiden-hair, Pauls Be-

Betony, Mousear, Agrimony, Comfrey, Scabious, Bugle, red Bramble leaves, Pelitory of the wall, Marsh Mallows and Plantain, of each half a handful, then take one spoonful of French Barley, a stick of Liquorish sliced small, one handful of Raisins *Solis* stoned; boil all these softly in a pottle of running water to a quart, then take it from the fire, and put to it two ounces of Conserve of red Roses, stir them together, and let it run through a fine cloth, and keep it close stopt in a glass, and drink thereof bloodwarm every morning and evening twelve spoonfuls at a time, for two, three, or four weeks, more or less, as you see occasion, and finde ease or pain.

A Special Medicine for one that cannot swallow, although no inward Medicine can be taken for it.

Take the soiling of a Dog that is hard and white, powder it, and mingle it well with English Honey, spread it thick upon a linnen cloth, and hold it to the fire, and lay it all over the Throat down to the Channel bone, use fresh morning and evening, binde it hard to, and by Gods grace it will help.

To draw up the Uvula.

Take a new laid Egg, and roast it till it be blue, and then crush it between a cloth, and lay it to the crown of the head, and once in twelve hours lay new till it be drawn up.

A Purge for Children or Old men.

Take one spoonful of Spirit of Tartar prepared, with Sugarcandy and Rose-water, put it in a little broath, and give it either of them; it purgeth gently, it comforts the Heart, and expelleth Phlegm and Melancholy.

For a Noli me tangere.

Take the Hearb called Turnsol, cut it in small pieces, and put it in a bottle, and pour so much *Aqua vitæ* on it as will cover it four fingers, stop the bottle, and set it in the Sun ten dayes, and in the night in the Chimney corner, but not too near the fire; then pour of the *Aqua vitæ*, and keep it close, then calcine the dregs remaining in the bottle be-

between two calcining pots well luted, which will be done in a day, then put the calcined ashes into the said *Aqua vitæ*, and they will all dissolve. Keep this as a great treasure, and give one spoonful thereof to the party fasting, in white Wine, and wet a cloth in the said Liquor, and binde it on the sore place, and without fail it will dry it up. It helpeth also those that are troubled with the Gravel and Stone, given as aforesaid with white Wine: and it is very excellent for those that have the Dropsie, Palsie, or are taken with a Quartane Ague.

To make the Face fair, and for a stinking Breath.

Take the flowers of Rosemary, and seethe them in white Wine, with which wash your face; if you drink thereof, it will make you have a sweet breath.

For heat in the Face, redness and shining of the Nose.

Take a fair linnen cloth, and in the morning lay it over the grass, & draw it over till it be wet with dew, then wring it out into a fair dish, and wet the face therewith as soft as you please, as you wet it let it dry in, *May dew is the best.*

An Excellent Oyl to take away the Heat and Shining of the Nose.

Take 12 ounces of Gourd-seed, crackle them, and take out the kernels, peel off the skin, and blanch six ounces of bitter Almonds, and make an Oyl of them, and anoint the place grieved therewith: you must always take as much of the Gourd-seed as of the Almonds; use it often.

For Heat or Pimples in the Face

Take the Liverwort that groweth in the Well, stamp and strain it, and put the juyce into Cream, and so anoint your Face as long as you will, and it will help you. *Proved.* Also the juyce of Liverwort drunk in beer warm, is good for the heat of the Liver.

To take away Hair.

Take the shells of fifty two Eggs, beat them small, and still them with a good fire, and with the water anoint your self where you would have the hair off: Or else Cats dung that is hard and dryed, beaten to powder, and tempered with strong Vinegar, and anointed on the place.

Dr. Friers *Receipt for sweating in the face.*

Take a little handful of Penniroyal, and as much Cinquefoil, and seethe them in white Wine or Vinegar; if you take Vinegar, put a little to it when it is sodden; this done you must hold your head over it, and cast a sheet over your head, and keep in the air close as long as you can endure it, and so ten or twelve times a day.

An approved Medicine taught by Dr. Blacksmith *for the Cough.*

Take the roots of Folefoot, and dry them in an Oven, and powder them, then heat a tile red hot, and strew it thereupon, then set the bottom of a tunnel upon it and let the Patient receive the same morning and evening.

An approved Medicine for the same, by Doctor Blacksmith.

Take a pint of Hysop-water, and a quarter of a pound of Sugarcandy, a spoonful of Anniseed bruised, and a small stick of Liquorish sliced and bruised, put them together, and let them stand all night, boil it a quarter of an hour upon a fire; then strain, and take of it two or three spoonfuls at a time warm; you may take it at any time, best at night when you go to bed, or in the morning.

For the Kidneys swoln with cold, or other Accident.

Take the Oyls of Roses and Quinces, of each two drams, and warm them in a Sawcer or Porringer, and anoint the place therewith against the fire, lest you take could in the doing of it.

A

A Vomit for an Ague.

Take blue Lilly-roots sliced small and bruised, and steep it in as much Vinegar as will cover them, and when the Patient feels his fit coming, let him drink a draught of it in Ale, and keep him very warm while it worketh.

A restorative Bag for a cold or windy Stomach.

Take Rose leaves, Rosemary tops, and flowers, red Mints, and Borage flowers, of each one handful, warm them in a platter on a Chafing-dish of coals, and ever as you stir it, sprinkle it with Sack and Rose-water; and when it is as hot as can be, put it in a cloth or silk bag, and lay it to the bottom of the Stomach, as hot as can be endured, and keep your self from studying or musing, and it will comfort very much.

A Drink for cold Rhumes or Phlegms.

Take the roots of Fennil, Comfrey, Parsley and Liverwort, Harts-tongue, E 5 Mousear,

Mousear, Horehound, Sandrake, Maidenhair, Cinquefoil, Hysop, Bugloss, and Violet leaves, of each one handful, wash and dry them very clean, Raisins *Solis* eight ounces, Anniseeds four drams, Liquorish two drams, Elecampane-root two drams, half a pint of Barley washed and bruised; boil these in a pottle of fair water, until half the liquor be consumed, strain it, and put to it one quart of White or Rhenish Wine, and 1. ounce of Sugarcandy, and boil it again till half be consumed, take it from the fire, and when it is cold put it into a clean glass, and drink thereof every morning and evening a draught first and last, and by Gods grace it will make you well and sound. *Approved.*

For Rhume in the Throat

Make a Cap of brown paper, perfume it with Frankincense, and apply it hot to the head, then take the hard Eggs, and lay them hot to the Nape of the Neck, and anoint the Throat with Oyls of Rice and sweet Almonds, and lay your self to sweat and after sweating, mix Mell Rosarum, Syrup

Syrup of Mulberries, Plantain water together, and gargle the throat therewith. In want of the said Syrup use Woodbin water.

A Remedy for the Stone.

Take a quart of Milk, Ale and white Wine of each four ounces, make them into a clear Posset drink, the curd taken off; to which put Parsley-roots, Mallow leaves, and Pellitory of the wall, of each one handful, Water-Cresses one handful and a half, all small shred, two sprigs of Time, and Liquourish one ounce bruised, boil all together to the consumption of a quart, and take a draught thereof in the morning, or at any time before meat, sweetned with Sugar to your taste.

A Broth for the Cough of the Lungs devised by Dr. Brasdale, Dr. Atkinson, and Dr. Fryer for the Lord Treasurer.

Take one paper of the prepared China roots, and steep in six pints of fair water three hours, then boil it unto three pints in an earthen pipkin, then boil

boil a Chicken and one ounce of French Barley together in a Pipkin six or seven Walmes, and skim it, then put away the water, and put the Barley and the Chick to the China, with the China in the paper a little green Endive, twenty Raisins of the Sun stoned, a little crust of bread, and a little Mace, boil them together unto a pint and half, strain it, and let the party drink every day two draughts thereof, one in the morning fasting, and another at four a clock in the afternoon, use it as often as you see cause.

For a Burning or Scalding.

Take Alehoof one handful, the yolk of an Egg, and some fair water, stamp them, and strain it, and therewith wash the grieved place till the fire be out.

Or boil some Alehoof and Sheep Suet together with Sheeps Dung and Plantain leaves, till they come to a salve, and apply it.

To procure Sleep.

Bruise a handful of Annifeeds, and
steep

steep them in red Rose-water, and make it up in little bags, and binde one of them to each Nostril, and it will cause sleep.

To sharpen a sick mans Appetite, and to restore his Taste.

Take Wood or Garden Sorrel one handful, and boil it in a pint of white wine Vinegar till it be very tender, strain it out, and put to it Sugar two ounces, and boil it to a Syrup, and let the Patient take of it at any time.

A Comfortable Juleb for a Feaver.

Take Barley-water and White Wine, of each one pint, Whey one quart, put to it two ounces of Conserve of Barberries, and the juices of two Lemons, and two Oranges. This will cool and open the body and comfort it. If the Feaver be extream hot, take two white salt Herrings, slit them down the back, and binde them to the soles of the feet for twelve hours. In want of Herrings, take two Pigeons cut open, and so apply them.

A

A Receipt of the Right Honourable the Lord Sheffield, *for the Cough of the Lungs.*

Take of the distilled water of sweet Horehound one pint, and adde thereto to make a Syrup three quarters of a pound of fine white Sugarcandy finely beaten, mix these well together, and set them upon a quick Charcoal fire, then take some of the best English Liquorish, clean scraped and sliced, and put into it, and let it boil in the said Syrup; and when it seems half boiled, take three grains of Ambergreese reasonable well bruised, and put it into the syrup, and let it boil altogether, but let any scum that riseth upon it be taken away before; you must have a care that it boil not with much heat, by often cooling some of it with a spoon; when it comes to a little thickness (being cold) it is boiled sufficiently, else will it be all candy, and not syrup, while it is hot it must be strained through a fine cloth that is clean, before it be put in a glass.

For a Cough or stuffing in the Stomach.

Take Hysop water one pint, Muscadine one quart, four races of Ginger, and as much Liquorish sliced, two penniworth of Sugarcandy in powder, put all into a glass, and stop it close, and shake them well together, and let it intermix twenty four hours, and drink thereof morning and evening.

A Plaister for the Cholick.

Take Cammomil, Rue, Sage, and Wormwood, of each one handful, Wheaten Bran half a handful, cut the hearbs small, and boil all in good Vinegar till the Vinegar be consumed, then put it into a linnen bag, and lay it to the pained place as hot as can be endured, and when it is cold warm it again, and use it daily till you be well.

For the rising of the Mother.

Take Columbine-seed, and Parsnip-seed, of each three spoonfuls; beat them to fine powder, and boil them in a quart

quart of Ale to a pint, seething with it one handful of Sage cut small, strain it, and drink it off warm every morning and evening; especially when you feel pain. And take two ounces of Galbanum, spread it upon a cloth, and lay it upon the womans Navil.

A Drink for the Dropsie.

Take Polopodie of the Oak six ounces, Guajacum one ounce, the Bark of Guajacum three ounces, Saffafras four ounces, Sena six ounces, Anni-seed three ounces, Epithymum, Stechados, of each half an ounce, Raisins *Solis* stoned eight ounces, Hermodactyles three ounces, Agarick, Rhubarb, China root, of each half an ounce, Liquorish four ounces; put all these to steep a whole night in two galons of Ale, and six quarts of strong Wine, in the morning boil them two hours and a half, the pot being close stopt, then strain it being cold, and give the Patient thereof three times a day, half a pint at a time, *viz.* at six in the morning, and at nine after that, and at three in the afternoon. Boil the remnant in the
strain-

strainer in strong Ale as before, and drink this second liquor at meals as often as you will. You must keep a drying diet of Roast meat every day, and sup betimes, but drink no other liquors whatsoever but these two.

For a Tympany or Water in ones Body, and for the fulness of the Stomach.

Take red Fennil and still it, and take thereof in the morning fasting a spoonful or two, and in the evening or any time of the day, when you feel your self not well: by Gods Grace this will help you.

For a Stich in the Side, proved.

Take a pretty quantity of Oats, and boil them in Sack, till they have dried up the sack, and then put them in a cloth, and lay it as hot as you can endure it to your side, and this will help.

A Receipt of Hearbs that are to be boiled in broth, according to Dr. Atkins opinion.

Take Tamarisk, Lettice, Borrage, Bug-

Bugloss, Rosemary tops, sweet Marjoram, Time, Succory, Parsley and Fennil, of each a pretty quantity, and when the body is costive, leave out some hearbs, and put in onely Tamarisk, Borage, Bugloss, Lettice, Succory, Parsley, Fennil, Betony.

Another by Mr. Francis Cox.

Take the Roots of Sparagus and Eringoes, of each three or four; cut off the length of a finger and sliced, Maiden-hair, Tamarisk, Harts-tongue, of each like much, Betony twice as much, as any of the rest, bind these and the roots together, take also large whole Mace two or three flakes, a quarter of a Nutmeg quartered; take then a young Cock, dress him, and slice him, and cut his flesh, and so boil him until he be sod all to pieces, but let not the Hearbs boil too long in the broth, but when they have given a pretty taste to it, take them out, and let the rest boil till the Chick be all in pieces; then beat the flesh of him with Dates in a stone Mortar, and strain it with the liquor, until you have all the taste

taste thereof in the liquor, then clarifie this broth with whites of Egs as you do a Jelly, and then use it; this broth will strengthen the back, and have respect to the Spleen.

A Preservative against the Plague.

Take one handful of Roses, Betony, and small Fellon, two handfuls of Scabious, of Dragon, Sage, Sorrel, Rue, Bramble leaves, and Elder leaves, of each one handful, Bole Armoniack as big as an apple, Saffron the weight of eight pence, yellow Sanders one ounce, Sugarcandy two ounces, all beaten into powder distil these together; take three spoonfuls thereof, and of Treacle or Mithridate the quantity of a bean, and mingle it with the water, and drink thereof when you are faint.

Oxymel Compositum.

Take pure Honey a pottle, White Wine Vinegar a pint and a half, five Parsley, five Fennil, five Smallage roots the pith taken out, the roots of Knacholm two ounces, Sparagus one ounce, Smallage

lage seed four ounces, shred the roots, and bruise the seeds, and steep them in three quarts of Conduit water for four and twenty hours, and after boil it all to one quart, strain it, and adde the Honey clarified and boil it therein, then put to the Vinegar, and let it boil gently to the thickness of a Syrrup, one spoonful whereof taken every morning fasting, cutteth and divideth all gross humours, it purgeth the Liver, Spleen, Reins, and opens all obstructions, it moveth Urine, and provoketh sweat.

A Purging Dyet-drink, the Proportion for four Gallons.

Take Sarsaparilla four ounces, Sena six ounces, Polypodie of the Oak six ounces, Rhubarb twelve drams, Sassafras roots two ounces, Agarick one ounce, Sea Scurvey-grass a peck, Fennil, Caroway and Aniseed, of each half an ounce, Cloves and Ginger, of each one ounce, wilde Radish, and white Flower de Luce roots, of each two ounces, Water-cresses and Brook-lime, of each eight handfuls, slice such of these as are to be sliced, and

and beat those that are to be beaten in a Mortar, and put them in a Canvas bag, and let it stand eight dayes in a Rundlet of four galons of ten shillings beer, a little lower then the middle of the beer, and so tun it. Take thereof in the Spring and Fall three or four dayes together in manner following, every morning at six a clock fasting, take half a pint cold, and use some exercise after it till you be warm, and fast till nine a clock; then take such another draught, and fast one hour after it, then take some thin warm broth, and keep a good diet at meals, eating no Sallads or Flegmatick meats: after dinner at three a clock take thereof another half pint, thus do for three or four dayes in the same manner. This will purge gently, clear the blood and inward parts, and prevent diseases. If you please, you may put to the above said Ingredients two handfuls of Maidenhair.

The Countess of Worcesters *Medicine for the Green Sickness approved.*

Take a pint of Malsey, and 2. handfuls of Currans clean washed, and put them together

gether, also take a little Wormwood, and a little crop or two of Red Mint, either green or dryed, and lay it in the Malmsey over night, and in the morning eat a spoonful or two of the Currans fasting, and walk after it, eating nothing in an hour; use this twelve dayes together, and if you shall see cause, also take Wormwood and warm it between two Tyles, and put it in a cloth, and lay to the stomach when you go to bed, and so fresh every night. Proved by the Lady *Worcester*.

A Diet Drink for a *Fistula*, or for a Body full of gross Humours.

Take Sarsaparilla, Sassafras, the Wood and Bark of Oak roots, of each four ounces cut small, Agrimony, Coltsfoot, Scabious, of each four handfuls, Marsh Mallow Roots half a handful, Betony, Ladies Mantle, Sinacle, Columbine roots of each one handful, shread the Hearbs and Roots small, and boil them all in three galons of Spring water, or two galons, then strain them through a Cullender, and put thereto one galon of clear water, and boil it to

a

Physical and Chyrurgical Receipts.

a galon and an half, and strain it again till all the moisture be out, put thereto a pottle of good white Wine, and a pint and half of good Honey, and boil it softly, scum it very clean; take it off the fire, and put to six drams of Rhubarb sliced small, and two ounces of Sena, and keep it in a stone vessel close covered, and drink thereof at five a clock in the morning, and at four a clock in the afternoon, till half of it be wasted; afterwards let the Patient drink thereof every morning a draught, and dress the Fistula with the green salve, and this will cure it. *wch see pag. 117.*

When this Drink is made as above-said, let it stand three dayes, onely shaking it together twice or thrice a day. It is fit to be drunk at three dayes end. In the time of taking it, all Fish, white meats, fruit, wine, anger and passion must be avoided.

For one that hath no speech in Sickness.

Take the juyce of Sage, or Pimpernel, and put it in the patients mouth, and by the grace of God it shall make him speak.

A Water good for Lightness of the Head, and the aforesaid.

Take the flowers of single White Primroses, and still them, and drink of the water, and that is good for the lightness of the head; and for bringing of the speech again, mingle therewith the like quantity of Rosemary-flower-water, and Cowslip-water, and the same will restore the speech again.

Sir Edward Boustwards *precious Oyntment for Aches in the Bones or Sinews that come of cold Causes.*

Take Wormwood, red Sage, the green and tender leaves and buds of Bayes and of Rue, of each one pound; chop them and beat them in a Mortar very small, put to them Mutton Suet well picked from the skins one pound and a half, and beat all well together, and put to them a pint and a half of good Oyl-Olive, or Neatsfoot Oyl, mix them all well together in an earthen pot, and set them in a warm Oven five hours, then take it out and strain it, and keep the Oyntment in an Earthen Pot,
anoint

anoint the grieved therewith well by the fire, and cover the place with black wool unwashed

Dr. Atkins. An excellent Medicine for the Jaundies.

Take of Rhubarb finely sliced the weight of a shilling, Red Dock roots sliced the weight of three shillings, one Nutmeg bruised grosly, and put them in a bottle of new beer, or any beer, the bottel being three quarts, or a pottle, let it be close stopped for three dayes, or two at least, and then begin to give him to drink thereof, every morning a draught next his heart, and about five a clock in the afternoon, drink this till his stool come yellow; if his body be loose with it, give him but onely in the morning: if he will not take this, give him two spoonfuls of the Syrup of Succory, with Rhubarb one morning, and every day after give him the weight of six pence of the powder after written, in drink or broth, or Aleberey next his heart for a week together.

Dr. Atkins Powder.

Take Earth-worms and flit them, and wash them with white Wine, then dry them in an Oven, and powder them, and put to every shilling weight of their powder, a groat weight of Ivory, and as much of Harts-horn scraped, and mingle them together, boil in his broth Parsley-roots and Fennil-roots, and a little Nutmeg; if he will not take this, give him every morning two spoonfuls of Oxymel Compositum alone, or in Beer, or else burn some Juniper, and take one ounce of the ashes, and put in an Hypocras bag, with a quarter of a Nutmeg beaten and run a pint of Rhenish Wine or White Wine through it four or five times, and let him every morning drink a draught of the Wine with Sugar.

An approved Medicine for the Yellow Jaundies.

Take the Peels of Barberries, and scrape off the outside of it, and take the inner peel of them, a quarter as much as one may hold in their hand, a small Reasin of Turmerick grated very small, four or five blades of English Saffron to be dried and beaten very small, then put all together, and boil in a pint of Milk or Posset drink, untill it be very bitter; then strain it, and drink every morning fasting, and at night when you go to bed, nine dayes together, and by the grace of God it will help you; Or else you may lay it a steep in strong Ale or Beer twenty four hours, and then drink a quantity of it, as you should the other; and if it be bitter, you may put a little Sugar to sweeten it.

To make Oyl of Excester.

Take Sage two handfuls, one of Time, one of the wild Vine, two of Hysop, one of Saint Johns Wort, two of Bay leaves, one of Goose-grass, two of Rosemary, one of Letterwood, two of Penniroyal, two of Cammomil, two of Lavender, two of White Lillies, two of Dragon leaves, two of Rue, two of Wormwood, two of Mints, one of Sweet Marjoram, one of Pellitory of Spain, one of Feaverfew, one of Angelica, one of

Betony,

Betony, stamp well these hearbs, and put them into a great pottage pot, and boil them in two quarts of running water till the water be consumed, then put to it two quarts of Cowslip flowers that have been steeped in Oyl Olive four weeks, and have been kept in the Sun all that time, and two quarts of White Wine, and also two quarts of Oyl Olive, boil them together one or two hours, till you think it almost dry, then strain in the Oyl from the hearbs, and put it into a glass, and blow the uppermost of the Oyl into the glass, for the very bottom is not so good.

A Medicine for the Worms.

Take a little fresh Butter and Honey, melt it, and anoint therewith the childe from the Stomach to the Navil, then take powder of Mirrhe, and strew it upon the place so anointed, cover it with a brown paper, and binde a cloth over it, and so anoint the childe three nights one after another. This Mirrhe is also good to swallow in a morning for shortness of breath, and to chew it in th mouth for Rhumes.

A Powder for the winde in the body.

Take Anniseed, Caroway-seed, Jet, Amber-greese, red Coral, dried Lemon or Orange peels, new laid Egg shels dried, Dates stones, pillings of Goose-horns, of Capons and Pigeons, dried Horse-radish-roots, of each half a scruple in fine powder well mixed, and take half a scruple thereof every morning in a spoonful of Beer or white Wine.

To make Oyl of Eggs.

Take twelve yolks of Eggs, and put them in a pot over the fire, and let them stand till you perceive them to grow black, then put them in a press, and press out the Oyl. This Oyl is good for all manner of burnings and scaldings whatsoever.

To make Oyl of Mustard seed.

Take two pounds of Mustard seed, and four pounds of Oyl Olive, grinde them together, and let them so stand nine dayes, and then stir it well, and keep in boxes. This Oyl is good for the Palsie, Gout, Itch, &c.

To make Oyl of Fennel.

Take a good quantity of Fennel, and and put it between two Iron Plates, and make them very hot in the fire, then press out the Liquor. This Oyl will keep a great while: It is good for the Tissick, and for Burnings or Scaldings.

To make Oyl of Rue.

Cut Rue leaves small, and put them into a pot with some Oyl Olive, and let them stand twelve dayes, then boil them till they be wasted to the third part, then strain it, and keep it close. This Oyl is good to keep away all causes of Pestilences in man, woman, or childe.

To make Oyl of Cammomil.

Stamp a good quantity of Cammomil flowers in a Mortar, put them in a pot with some Oyl Olive, and let them

them stand twelve days, then boil it a little on the fire, then take it off, and press it out hard, and put the Juyce into glasses, and put to them more Cammomil flowers stamped small, and let them stand for your use.

A Soveraign Medicine for a Fistula.

Take pure Rosin one pound, Sheep Suet the bigness of a great Egg, or somewhat more in Winter, and set them on a fire in a pot, till it be ready to boil, then pour it in a pan of cold water, and work it with your hands rubbed with Butter, till it become so small as Pack thred, scrape it on a cloth, and spread it thin, then cut it out small and narrow, & when you use it, roll it up small like tents.

The Powder.

Take an Ox horn, and steep it nine dayes in water, shift every day into fresh water; then take it out, and fill it full of black Soap, and fry it over the fire in a Frying-pan, and the horn will melt away and burn to powder; dip the end of ten tents in this powder.

The water.

Take Allum and white Copperas of each half a pound, beat them into fine powder, and mix them well together, and put them in an earthen pot, and let them boil on a soft fire till they be hard, and will boil no longer, then beat them to powder. Two spoonfuls will make a galon of water, and one spoonful will make a pottle, but let the water seethe first; then take it off, and at first sprinkle a little of the powder lest it flame up, and after the rest wet a fair cloth, and dress the sore twice a day. If green Copperas be used, two pound must be put to one pound of Allum. When the sore is dressed, it must be tented as aforesaid if need require, and lay on a cloth still wet in the said water. As the water comes hot from the fire, put in one spoonful of the said powder by degrees.

A special Medicine for a Looseness.

Burn three Nutmegs to ashes in the flame of a wax candle, and when they are throughly burnt, rub them to powder, and mix it with the like quantity of of Bean-flower and Cinnamon finely beaten and fearfed, then make up into a paste with the white of an Egg, and a little red Wine, and make the paste into small round pills fit for swallowing, and dry them hard in a clean fire, and when you take them, drink a little red wine after it.

For an Uncomb or Sore Finger.

Shred one handful of Smallage very small, and put to it one spoonful of Honey, the yolk of an Egg, and a little Wheat flower to make it thick, then spread it on a cloth, and lay it to the sore twice a day.

For the same in young Children, or any other in the beginning.

Take Celandine, and bruise it well between your hands, and binde to your Navil, and the soles of your feet; hang it once in twenty four hours till they be well.

F 5

A Medicine for the Purples, proved.

Take Purple Silk, and shred it as small as you can, and put it into a spoon, and put a little Ale or Beer unto it lukewarm, and so take it, and drink after it a little, and so do five mornings together, and fast an hour after it.

Dr. Twines *Almond Milk.*

Take a pot of water when it is boiled, and stood to be clear, then boil therein Violet leaves, Strawberries the whole hearb with the root, of each a pretty handful, Sorrel a good root all well washed, a crust of white Bread, Raisins of the Sun stoned two ounces, boil all these from a pottle to a quart, and with fifty Almonds blanched, and thirty Pompion Kernels, all well beaten, draw an Almond Milk, sweetened with good Sugar to your liking, and drink a good draught thereof morning and evening towards the quantity of a pint.

Dr. Blacksmiths *Almond Milk.*

Take of the roots of Ruscus Gramen, Sparagus and Succory, each three drams, Barley prepared half a handful, of the leaves of Mallows, Violets, five leaved Grass, Strawberries, Borage, Bugloss, Maiden-hair, of each half a handful, sliced Liquorish two drams; boil all these in three pints of fair running water to a quart or less: then take the weight of a French Crown of the Kernels of each of the three cold seeds, and beat them with a few Almonds, and white Rose water and Sugar, and make Almonds Milk.

Dr. Atkins *excellent Receipt of Almond Milk to cool and cleanse the Kidneys.*

Take a pint and quarter of Barley-water, and in that boil Althea, Iringus, Gramen and Sparagus roots each a French Crowns weight, Strawberries, and five leaved Grass, both leaves and roots, each a few, boil them till the Barley-water be but a pint, then strain out the Barley-water, and take a French Crown

Crowns weight, a piece of the four cold seeds, and peel off the husks, then beat the seeds with the Almonds, and strain them forth together with the Barley water, and put to it a little Rose-water and Sugar, and make it an Almond Milk.

A Receipt for the Stone

Take a galon of new Milk, Wilde Time, Saffafras, Pellitory of the Wall, Philipendula roots, Saxifrage, of each one handful, Parsley, leaves two handfuls, three or four Radish-roots, and as many Parsley-roots, Annifeeds one ounce, cut and flit the roots, bruife the hearbs and feeds, and put them to infuse in the milk a whole night, the next morning diftil it in a Rose diftillatory. Take ten or twelve fpoonfuls of the water, and as much White or Rhenifh Wine, a little Sugar, and a fliced Nutmeg. It is very good every full and change of the Moon to take morning and evening, to prevent fickness, and at any time if need require.

For the Green sickness.

Take Aloes and Rhubarb, of each four ounces finely beaten and searsed, prepared Steel four drams; mix these together with Claret Wine, and make them into twenty seven pills, and take every morning in three of them, using exercise till all be gone, and drink after them at each time a glass of Claret wine.

For any sore Breasts or Paps.

Take a pottle of running water, Sage two good handfuls small minced, and a quantity of Oatmeal-greats small beaten; boil all these to the thickness of White Bread dough, but let it not burn to, then put to it three spoonfuls of Honey, and a little Saffron; stir it well together, and boil it to a quart somewhat stiff. This Pultess will break and heal it soon, and draw away the pain without breaking. It will cure any sore Breast or Pap, if it be not a Canker or Fistula.

A Syrrup lasting many years, good for Swounding and Faintness of Heart, it comforteth the weak Brain and Sinows, it may be used as much as half a nut once at your pleasure.

Take Borage, Bugloss, white Endive, one little handful, of Rosemary-flowers, Time, Hysop, Winter Savory, of each one little handful; break these between your hands, and seethe them in three quarts of water to three pints, then strain it, and put to it a pint of good Malmsey, one ounce of whole Cloves, powder of Cinnamon half an ounce, powder of Ginger a quarter of an ounce, one Nutmeg in powder, Sugar half a pound or more, let them seethe upon a soft fire, well stirred for burning to, until it come to the thickness of Honey, then take it up, and let it cool, and put it in pots or glasses at your pleasure. Prescribed by Dr. *Twine*.

An approved Medicine for a woman in Labor to make, come, & prove safe deliverance.

Take powder of Cinnamon one dram, powder of Amber half a dram finely beaten,

beaten, mingle it with eight spoonfuls of Claret Wine, and so let her drink it.

To Know how much Bezar Stone must be taken when one is heart sick.

Take Bezer Stone the weight of three Barley corns, or five at a time, once in six or ten hours; and give it in a spoon with Carduus, Bean-water, Borage, or Bugloss, Ale or Beer.

Doctor Stevens excellent water, wherewith he cured many Diseases following.

Take one galon of Gascoign Wine, Ginger, Gallingal, Cammomil, Nutmegs, Grains of Paradise, Cloves, Annifeeds, Caroway-seeds, of each one dram, then take Sage, Mint, red Roses, Time, Pellitory, Rosemary, Penniroyal, Montanum, Cammomil, Babin, Harts-tongue, Lavender, Avance, of each a handful, bray the spices small, and let stand so twelve hours, stirring it divers times; then still it in a Limbeck, and keep the first by it self, for it is best; then will there

there come a second water which is good, but not so good as the first, for it is fainter. The vertues of this water is, to comfort the Vital Spirit greatly, and preserve the youth of man or woman, and helps the inward diseases that come of cold, helpeth the shaking of the Palsie, and cureth contractions of Sinnews, it strengthneth the Marrow in the bones, it helpeth the conception of Women that are barren, it killeth Worms in the body, and cureth the cold Gout, and Tooth-ache, and it helpeth the Stone in the bladder, and the pain in the Reins of the Back, and will make one seem young a long time; one spoonful of this *Aqua vitæ* shall do more good to a man that is sick, then four spoonfuls of any other; and this *Aqua vitæ* shall be better if it stand in the Sun all Summer long.

For the Falling Sickness.

Take half a peck of Peony roots, cleanse, rub, wash and stamp them, and as you stamp them, put in Sherry Sack, let them be beaten very small, and then put to them a pottle of Sherry Sack, stir

stir all well together, and let it stand close covered twenty four hours, then pour of the clearest into bottles, and take thereof a little draught every change of the Moon, for three mornings, one morning after another.

A Pultess to break a Bile or Impostume.

Take Sorrel one handful, twelve Figs quartered, half a pint of Sorrel juyce; boil and break these together till it be very tender, and put to it some Wheat flower, and when it is well boiled, put to it a good piece of Butter, and lay it warm to the place twice a day, till it be drawn enough.

A Remedy for Worms in Children.

Take one spoonful of juyce of Lemons, powdered Saffron half a scruple, and a little Sugar; and give this same quantity to the patient three mornings together.

For Worms. Dr. Wetherborn.

Take Rhubarb one dram, Wormwood

wood half a dram, Corralline one scruple, Currans one good handful, beat them all to a Conserve, and mix it with Syrup of Violets, to an Electuary, and give a childe the quantity of a Walnut thereof every other morning fasting.

An Oyntment to heal any bruise or wound.

Take Sage, Self-heal, Smallage, Southernwood, Plantain, Time, Ribwort, Rue, Parsley, Marigold leaves, Mercury, Wormwood, Betony, Scabious, Valerian, Cumfrey, Lions-tongue, Buck-horn, of each one handful; wash them clean, and put them into a Sieve to drain all night, and when they are dry, chop them very small, and put to them two pounds of unwashed Butter well beaten, then boil it till half be consumed, then strain it into the pot you mean to keep it in. It is also good for swollen Breasts. *May* is the best time to make it in.

For a Bruise in a womans breast that is hard swoln.

Take Wood-lice, and dry them between papers before the fire, and make them into fine powder, whereof take as much as will lie on a three pence in a spoonful of Gout Ale: do thus first and last for three weeks together, and after you may take twice a week, till you finde the Breast well. But you must be sure to keep a white Cotton fried in Goose grease to it constantly, though you leave taking the said powder, until you finde the Breast cured. This hath cured Breasts that should have been cut off.

A Medicine for a childe that cannot hold his or her Water.

Take the Navil string of a child which is ready to fall from him, dry it and beat it to powder, and give it to the patient childe Male or Female in two spoonfuls of small Beer to drink fasting in the morning.

A. R. C.

Shred two handfuls of Rosemary flowers, and boil them in a quarter of a pint of *Aqua vitæ* a little together. At night when you go to bed, and in the morning you must have two little pieces of white Cotton, and take some of this liquor, and set it on the embers in a dish, and put in one of the pieces of Cotton, and when it is hot, wring out the liquor, and lay it to the grief. Do thus three times evening and morning, keeping the last piece of Cotton to the grief all night, and so all day.

An Electuary for the Liver.

Take Cichory roots, wash and rub them very dry in a cloth, then slit them and take out their pith, and cut them in small pieces, of these roots thus ordered take eight ounces, and beat them small in a Mortar, and put to them two ounces of Currans well washed and dry rubbed in a cloth, and beat them well together, put one ounce of the best grated Rhubarb, and half a pound

pound of double refined Sugar, beaten to powder, and beat all well together in the Mortar to the consistence of a well formed Electuary, and keep in a galley-pot for your use close covered. Take as much thereof as a Walnut in the morning fasting, and as much at four a clock in the afternoon.

A purging Ale for the Liver.

Take Scurvy-grass six handfuls, Brooklime, Water-cresses, of each three handfuls, Agrimony, Speed-wel, Liverwort, of each two handfuls, Fennel and Parsley roots, of each three ounces, Horse-radish two ounces, Monks Rhubarb one pound, all well picked, washed and bruised; then put to them Sena five ounces, Polypody of the Oak four ounces, Nutmegs bruised two ounces, Fennel-seed bruised one ounce, Liquorish slit and bruised two ounces, Sassafras cut small three ounces: put all these in a bag or boulter, and hang it in five or six galons of second Ale, and after five dayes infusion, drink thereof half a pint every morning fasting, and walk upon it.

A Medicine for the Stone.

Take the Pulp of Cassia Fistula newly drawn one ounce and a half, Rhubarb in powder one dram and a half, Venice Turpentine seven drams, Liquorish half a dram, Species of Diatragacanthum Frigidum one scruple, mix them well together with a sufficient quantity of Marsh Mallows, and take thereof in the morning fasting the quantity of a Walnut, and drink after it a good draught of posset drink; use it three mornings at every new Moon.

For the Whites and Heats in the Back.

Take three or four Nutmegs, and put them into the middle of a brown loaf, set it in an Oven, and when it is baked take out the Nutmegs, and every morning for nine dayes one after another, beat the white of a new laid Egg to water, then put to it of Plantain and red Rose-water, of each four spoonfuls, and grate into it some of the said Nutmegs, and sweeten it with a little Sugar, and drink it off.

Syrup of Ale for the same Disease.

Take a galon of new Ale-wort of the first tunning, and hang it over the clear fire in an Iron Pot, and scum it till no more will rise, and when it is boiled to a pint take it off, and put it into an earthen pot with a cover, and take a little thereof on a Pen-knifes point every morning and evening.

An excellent artificial Balsam.

Take Conduit-water and Oyl Olive, of each one quart, Turpentine four ounces, liquid Storax six ounces; put them in a Bason, and let them stand together all night, the next day melt half a pound of Bees-wax on the fire, and put to it Rosemary, Bayes and sweet Marjoram, of each one handful shred small, and also Dragons blood, and Mummey, of each one ounce made small, and let them boil in the wax a while; then put into the Bason Oyl of Saint Johns-wort and Rose-water, of each two ounces, and boil it together a little more, then put in some natural Balsam

sam and red Sanders pulverised, and let it boil a little, then strain it into a bason, and when it is cold make a hole in it with a knife to let out the water, & so dissolve it on the fire, and put it up for your use.

The Vertues and Operations of this Balsam are.

1. It is good to cure any wound inward, if inward, squirt it in, or apply it with a tent: if outward, anoint the place.

2. It healeth any burning or scalding, bruise or cut, being therewith anointed, and a linnen cloth or lint dipped therein laid to the place warm.

3. It takes away any pain or grief, that comes of cold and moisture in the bones or sinews, anointing the place grieved with this Oyl heated, and a warm cloth laid on it.

4. It cureth the headache, onely anointing the temples and nostrils therewith.

5. It is good for the Winde Cholick, or Stitch in the sides, applied thereunto warm with hot clothes four mornings together every morning a quarter of an ounce.

And many other cures it doth, &c.

To make the Green Oyntment.

Take Rue and Sage, of each one pound, Bay leaves and Wormwood, of each half a pound, Melilot, the Hearb and Flowers of Cammomil, Spike, Rosemary, red Rose leaves, Saint Johns-wort, and Dill, of each one handful, chop them first very small, then stamp them, and put thereto the like weight of Sheeps Suet chopt very small, and stamp them all in a stone Mortar to one substance, that all be green and no Suet appear. Then put it into a large earthen pan, and pour on it five pints of pure and sweet Oyl Olive, and work them together with your hands to one substance; then cover the pan with paste close, that no air enter, and let it stand seven dayes, then open it and put it in a fresh pan; and set it on a soft fire alwayes stirring it till the hearbs begin to grow parched, then strain it into a fresh pan, to which put the Oyls of Roses, Cammomil, white Lillies, Spike and Violets, of each one ounce, stir them well together, and keep it in a glass close stopt for your use.

An Electuary for the passion of the Heart.

Take Damask Roses half blown, cut off their whites, and stamp them very fine, and strain out the Juyce very strong, moisten it in the stamping with a little Damask-Rose-water, then put thereto fine powder Sugar, and boil it gently to a thin Syrup; then take the powders of Amber, Pearl and Rubies, of each half a dram, Ambergreese one scruple, and mingle them with the said syrup, till it be somewhat thick, and take a little thereof on a knifes point morning and evening.

A drink for a hot Feaver.

Take Spring-water and red Rose-water, of each one pint and a half, the juyce of three Lemons, and white Sugarcandy one ounce, and mix them together, and give the Patient thereof six or eight spoonfuls at a time often in a day and night, until the unnatural heat be extinguished

For the Cholick.

Take equal portions of Honey and Wine, put them on a fire, and put thereto ground Wheat-meal, and a pretty quantity of bruised Cummin-seeds, and as much Sorrel, boil all together for a pretty while, then put them into a linnen bag, and apply it to the belly as a plaister. Or take a pretty bundle of Time, and boil it with a little slice of Ginger in a pint of Malmsey til the third part be wasted, and drink thereof as warm as you can.

For stopping of the Urine.

Take the shels of quick Snails, wash them and dry them clean, and beat them into fine powder; whereof take a pretty quantity in White Wine, or thin broth.

For the Stone in the Kidneys.

Take a pottle of new Ale, and as much Rhenish Wine, and put into it two whole Lemons sliced with the peels and all, and put to them one Nutmeg beaten, and two handfuls of Scurvey-grafs beaten and ſtrained into the Ale, and half a penniworth of grains of Paradiſe bruiſed; put all together in a little ſtand with a cover, and after three dayes drink of it with a taſte. It is alſo good againſt the winde Cholick, proceeding from the Stone.

To make Hair grow thick.

Take three ſpoonfuls of Honey, and a good handful of Vine ſprigs that twiſt like Wire, and beat them well, and ſtrain their juyce into the Honey, and anoint the bald places therewith.

For the Rhume or Cough in the Stomach.

Take a pint of Malmſey or Muſcadine, and boil it in five ounces of Sugarcandy till it come to a Syrup, and in the latter end of the boiling put to it five ſpoonfuls of Horehound diſtilled water, and ſo ſuck it from a Liquoriſh ſtick bruiſed at the end. Uſe this onely to bed-ward.

For the Sciatica.

Take a pound of yellow Wax, six spoonfuls of the juyce of Marjoram and red Sage, two spoonfuls of the juyce of Onions, of Anniseeds, Cloves, Frankincense, Mace and Nutmegs, of each one penniworth, and as much Turpentine; boil these together to the consistence of a Salve, and so apply it.

For the Piles.

Roast quick Snails in their shels, pick out their meat with a pin, and beat them in a Mortar with some powder of Pepper to a salve; then take the dried roots of Pilewort in powder, and strew it thin on the Plaister, and apply it as hot as you can suffer it.

To procure Sleep.

Chop Cammomile and crumbs of brown bread small, and boil them with White Wine Vinegar; stir it well and spread it on a cloth and binde it to the soles of the feet as hot as you can suffer

fer it You may adde to it dried red Rose-leaves, or red Rose-cakes with some red Rose-water, and let it heat till it be thick, and binde some of it to the Temples, and some to the Soles of the feet.

A good Purge.

Take Diacatholicon and Syrrup of Roses Laxative, of each one ounce, mix them well together in a penny pot of white Wine, and drink it warm early in the morning. This purgeth Choler, Flegm, and all maner of watry humors.

For a Fellon in a Joynt.

Dry Bay-salt, and beat it into powder, and mix it with the yolk of an Egg, and apply it to the grieved place in the beginning, before the Fellon be broken: but if he be first broken, then take the juyce of Groundsel, the yolk of an Egg, a little Honey and Rye-flower, mix them well together, and so apply it.

To heal a fresh Wound with speed.

Take the leaves of Columdine Nettles, Plantain, Ribwort, wilde Tarras, Wormwood, red Roses, Betony, Violets, of each one handful; wash them clean, and beat them well with the White of an Egg, and strain out the juyce through a cloth, to which juyce put the quantity of two Walnuts of Honey, and half an ounce of Frankincense; stir them well together, and put it in a box, and use it Plaister-wise. Or take Rosin, Wax, fresh Butter, Barrows grease well tried, of each a little quantity, oyl them well, and put it into a bason of cold water, and work it with your hands into little rolls, spread it on a cloth, and apply it. If the wound be deep, tent it with lint.

For the pricking of a Needle or Thorn.

Take boulted Wheat-flower, and temper it with red Wine, boil them together to the thickness of a Salve; and lay it on so hot as you can suffer it. This will open the hole, draw out the filth and ease the pain.

For to kill a Corn.

Take of the bigness of a Walnut of Ale yeast that is hard, and sticks to the tub side, put to it a little dried salt finely powdered; work them well together, and put it in a close box, make a plaister of some of it, and binde it to the Corn.

For Bruises, Swellings, broken Bones.

Take Brook-lime, Chickweed, Mallows, Smallage, Groundsel, of each one handful, stamp them with a little Sheeps tallow, Swines grease, and Copin, put thereto wine dregs, and a little Wheat Bran; stir them well together over the fire till they be hot, so apply it to the place grieved.

For Burning or Scalding.

Take Goose dung, and the middle bark of an Elder tree, fry them in *May* Butter, strain them, and therewith anoint the burnt or scalded place.

To help Deafness.

Take a piece of Rye dough the bigness of an Egg, and of that fashion, bake it dry in an Oven, cut off the end, and with a knife cut out the paste and make it hollow, then put into it a little Aqua Composita, and stir it; and so hot as you can endure it, apply it to the deaf ear till it be cold, you must keep your head very warm. If both ears be grieved, make two of them, and use those three times.

For the Cholick.

Take half a sheet of white paper, anoint it all over with Oyl Olive, and strew thereon gross Pepper, and so lay it to the belly from the navil downward.

For the yellow Jaundies.

Take Pimpinel, Groundsel, Sheebroom, with the tops, of each one handful, boil them in a quart of Ale till half be consumed, then divide it into three draughts, and take it morning and evening.

For the Bloody Flux.

Take Bean-flower, mingle it with Malmsey, and make a paste thereof, and bake it in an Oven like a Cake, but not too hard, and lay it upon the Navel of the Belly as hot as can be suffered, and wet it over with Malmsey, and keep it warm. It will help in three dayes.

A Drink to drive the Plague from the Heart.

Take a great Onion, cut off the top of it, and take out so much of the Core, as the bigness of a Walnut, which hole fill up with Treacle, put on the top again, and wrap the Onion in a piece of brown or gray paper, roast it throughly, and peel it, and trim it finely, and put it in a clean linnen cloth, and strain it hard into three Porringers, and drink the juyce so strained out: for it hath been found most excellent by often proof, not onely for the expulsion of the Plague, but also for the eradicating of all poison and venome.

The onely Receipt against the Plague.

Take three pints of Muscadine, and boil therein a handful of Sage, and a handful of Rue, until a pint be wasted. Then strain it, and set it on the fire again. Then put thereto a penniworth of Long Pepper, half an ounce of Nutmegs all beaten together. Then let it boil a little, and put thereto three penniworth of Treacle, and a quarter of the best Anglica water you can get: keep this as your life above all worldly Treasure. Take of it alwayes warm both morning and evening a spoonful or two, if you be already infected, and sweat thereupon, if not a spoonful in the morning, and half a spoonful at evening in all the Plague time, under God trust to this, for there was neither Man, Woman nor Childe by this deceived.

This is not onely for the Common Plague, which is called the Sickness, but for the Small Pocks, Measles, and Surfeits, and divers other Diseases.

A good

A good Almond Milk for the bloody Flux.

Take Mutton and boil it in fair water, and scum it very clean, then put to it a handful of Borage leaves, as much Prunes, some Cinnamon and whole Mace, the upper crust of a Manchet; boil all these well till their strength be gone into the broth, then strain it through a Cullender, then take Jordan Almonds, and parch them as you do Pease, and let them boil two or three Walms, then strain them through a cloth, and season it well with Sugar and a little Salt, and let the Patient drink thereof at all times of the day. It is very Medicinal.

To take fish by Angling.

Take Assa Fetida, Camphire, Aqua vitæ and Oyl Olive, bray them together till they come to a soft Oyntment, then box it, and anoint your baits therewith.

For an Ache or Swelling.

Take Oatmeal, Sheeps suet, and
black

black Soap, of each four ounces, boil them in water till they be thick, make a plaister of it, and apply it to the grieved place hot.

For a Childes Navil that comes out with much crying.

Take Wax as it comes from the Bee-hive, let it not be altered, but onely strained from the Honey, then melt some of it in a Sawcer, and dip some black Sheeps Wool in it, and binde it to the Navil.

For Womens sore Paps or Breasts.

Take Bean-flowers two handfuls, Wheaten Bran, and powder of Fenugreek, of each one handful, one pound of white Wine Vinegar, three spoonfuls of Honey, three yolks of Eggs, boil all till they be very thick, and lay it warm to the Breast. This will both break and heal it. Chrush out the matter when you change the Plaister. Or take Oyl of Roses, Bean-flower, and the yolk of an Egg with a little Vinegar, set it on the fire till it be lukewarm.

warm and no more, then with a feather anoint the sore places.

For an Ague in Womens Breasts.

Take the leaves of Hemlock, fry them in sweet Butter, and as hot as may be suffered apply it to the Breasts, and lay a warm white Cotton on it, and in short time it will drive the Ague out of them.

To draw Rhume from the Eyes back into the Neck.

Take twenty Catharides, cut off their heads and wings, and beat their bodies into small powder, which put in a little linnen bag, and steep it all night in *Aqua vitæ* or Vinegar, and lay it to the Nape of the neck, and it will draw some blisters, which clip off, and apply to them an Ivy or Cabbage leaf, and it will draw the Rhume from the Eyes. Or roast an Egg hard, cut it in half and take out the yolk, and fill either side with beaten Cummin-seed, and apply it hot to the Nape of the Neck.

For a Canker in the mouth.

Take a pint of strong Vinegar, Roach Allum the bigness of a Walnut, as much English Honey as will sweeten it, and boil it in a skillet, put it up in a close stopt glass, warm a little of it in a Sawcer, and therewith wash the mouth often, and lay some lint wet in the same warm liquor upon the places.

To make a sweet Breath.

Take the dried flowers and tops of Rosemary, Sugarcandy, Cloves, Mace and Cinnamon, of each a like quantity dried and beaten into fine powder; then take a new laid Egg, and put of the powder into the Egg, and sup it off fasting in a morning; do so seven dayes one after another, and it will sweeten the breath.

For an old Sore Leg.

Take the whitest hard Soap you can get, scrape a quantity thereof into a Sawcer, put to it some Deer suet, and boil

boil them on the fire, then spread it on a clean linnen cloth, and lay it to the sore morning and evening, and in a short time it will heal.

For a Stitch in the Side.

Take a piece of white leavened bread, and toast it on both sides, then spread one side thereof with the best Treacle you can get, and cover it with a fine linnen cloth, and so lay it to the grieved place.

A most excellent Salve for a Wound.

Take a good quantity of the tops of Maiden or unset Hysop, shred them small, and beat them very small in a Mortar; then take Oyl Olive and clarified Honey, of each one spoonful, put thereto half a handful of Wheat-flower, compound them together cold, and make it up into a fine Salve, which use to the purpose aforesaid.

A Pultess to ripen any Bile or Impostume.

Take a Lilly root and roast it in the Em-

Embers in a brown paper, then take Figs and pound them small, and Fenugreek, and Linseed, of each a like quantity: when the Lilly root is roasted, pound it very well, then boil all therein new Milk from the Cow, till it be so thick that a spoon may stand upright in it, and stir it alwayes in the boiling, and put to it some Barrows grease and apply it to the place grieved.

To encrease Womans Milk.

Take Fennel-seeds bruised, and boil them well in Barley-water, whereof let wet Nurses and Suckling Women drink very often; in winter warm, in summer cold, and let them beware of drinking much strong Beer, Ale or Wine, for they are hot, and great driers up of Milk; and so are all Spices, and too much Salt or salt meat.

To keep Iron from Rusting.

Take Lead filed very small, and put so much Oyl Olive upon it, as will cover it in a pot, then make your Iron very clean first, and anoint the Iron with the
said

said Oyl, after it hath stood nine dayes, and it will never rust.

To make Golden Colour without Gold.

Take the juyce of Saffron flowers, when they are fresh on the ground, but if you cannot get them, then take Saffron dried and powdered, and put to it Yellow and Glistering Auripigment, that is scalie, and with the Gall of a Hare, or Pike fish, which is better, mix them together; then put them in a glass Vial close stopped, which set in a warm Dunghil for certain dayes, then take it out, and keep it for your use.

To make Golden Letters without Gold.

Take Auripigment one ounce, fine Crystal one ounce, beat them to powder severally, then mix them, and then temper them with the whites of Egs, and so write with it.

To make Silver Letters without Silver.

Take Tin one ounce, Quicksilver two ounces, melt them together; then
beat

beat them well with Gum-water; and so write with it.

To make the Face fair.

Take fresh Bean Blossoms, and distill them in a Limbeck, and with the water wash your face.

A Wound Drink.

Take Southernwood, Wormwood, Bugle, Mugwort, White bottle, Sanicle, Plantane, Dandelion, Cinquefoil, Ribwort, Wood Betony, Clary roots, Avens called Herb Bennet, Hawthorn buds, Agrimony, Oak leaves and buds, Bramble buds, wilde Angelica, Mints, Scabious, Strawberry leaves, Violet leaves, Comfrey, of each twenty handfuls; gather them in *May*, and dry them in a room without much fire, turn them often, that they may not become musty; and when they are dry, put them up in Canvas bags severally. Then take of these several hearbs so dried, of each three handfuls, and put them into two quarts of running water, and one quart of White Wine, boil them to three pints, strain the liquor from the hearbs, and

and put thereto one pint of Honey, which boil again, taking away the froth, then strain it, and keep it in glass bottle close stopped, and take thereof in the morning fasting, and at night last, two or three spoonfuls at one time. This water will not continue good above three or four weeks at the most. It cureth old sores, green wounds, Impostumes, Fistulas, and stancheth bleeding. Tent no wound, but search and cleanse it in a tent, and cover the place with a clean cloth. During the cure, the Patient must keep a spare diet, and abstain from Wine and strong Drink.

For Worms in *Children*.

Take three pound of Prunes, Sena one ounce and a half, sweet Fennel-seed one ounce and a half Rhubarb half an ounce; tie all these in a bag with a stone to it, and put them into a great quantity of water, then put the Prunes on the top, and let it stew six or seven hours, till the liquor be even with the Prunes; so drink of the liquor two or three spoonfuls, and eat of the Prunes in the morning fasting, and at four clock in the afternoon.

A Green Salve.

Take one pound of Butter, Bees-wax five ounces, Rosin one pound and a half, Frankincense four ounces, Oyl of Bayes two ounces, Deer suet one ounce and a half, Verdigreese one ounce and a half, boil the butter a little, then boil the Wax in it, and stir it now and then, take it off the fire, put in the Oyl of Bayes, set it on the fire again, then put in the Deer suet, and let it boil one walm, for if it have more it will turn black, and when it is off the fire, put in the Verdigreese powdered, then strain it into pots, and keep it for your use.

A Receipt for the Kings Evil, Fistula, sore Breasts, Legs, or other sores.

Take Samnil, Agrimony, Avens, wilde Bugle, red Dandelion, Wood Betony, Ribwort, Wilde Clary roots and leaves, Mugwort, Plantain, Wormwood and Bugle heaten and bruised, of each two handfuls, boil them in six quarts of white Wine until their vertue be extracted very softly, then with your

your hand squeeze all the juyce out of them into the Wine, then strain the liquor out, and set it on the fire, and clarifie it with so much Honey as will make it dainty, pleasant, and not sharp; then let it boil a little more, and when it is cold, put it in bottles close stopped, and it will last a year, whereof give the Patient six spoonfuls at a time, in the morning fasting, and at four a clock in the afternoon.

To ease Womens Child-bed throws that are taken with cold a week or two after their Delivery.

Take one or two spoonfuls of Oyl of sweet Almonds newly drawn, either in Posset drink, or in a Caudle warm morning and evening it will help.

For Womens sownding fits after delivery of Childe.

Take the powder of White Amber as much as will lie on a three pence, and give it in Mace Ale warm.

An

An approved Medicine to speed a Womans Delivery in difficult Travel, and to send out the after-burthen safely.

Take Cinnamon two drams and a half, one dram and a half of white Amber, Myrrhe two scruples, Castoreum one scruple, Borax half a scruple, Saffron five grains, powder and mix them, whereof give one dram at a time in white Wine and Sugar, and sweat after it. This hath been often tried with much good success.

An approved Medicine for the Megrum.

Take one spoonful and a half of the white of an Egg beaten very clear, white Wine Vinegar one spoonful, of Pepper and Frankincense, of each two drams powdered, and one spoonful of Honey, mix them with so much Wheat flower as will make it into paste, whereof make two plaisters, and lay them to the Temples of the head, and change it duly every morning and evening.

For to ease Head Pain.

Take red Rose leaves dried, mix them with Wheat-flowers, Vinegar, Oyl of Roses, and some Housleek, boil them till they be thick, spread it on a linnen cloth, and lay it to the Forehead and Temples, and it will ease the pain.

To cure a Shock Dog that hath the Mangie.

Take four ounces of Tar, mix it with some fresh grease, so as it may run; then put to it some Brimstone powder half a spoonful of Gun-powder powdered, and two spoonfuls of Honey, mix them well, and therewith anoint the Dog; in the summer time tie him in the hot Sun, that the Oyntment may soak into him, in the winter time lay him on thick fresh Hay, and there keep him that the heat of his body may heat and melt it. Thrice drssieng will cure him.

Dr. Goffes Receipt to preserve a Woman with childe from miscarrying, and abortion.

Take a Fillet of Beef half roasted hot from the fire, then take half a pint of Muscadine, Sugar, Cinnamon, Ginger, Cloves, Mace, Grains of Paradise and Nutmegs, of each half a dram, and make thereof a Sawce, then divide the Beef into two pieces, and wet them in the Sawce, and binde the one piece to the bottom of the womans belly, and the other to the reins of the back, as hot as may be suffered, and keep them on twenty four hours at the least, and longer if need be thereof.

For any Pain in the Stomach.

Cut a piece of new Scarlet in the shape of a Heart, put it in a pewter dish, and wet it with strongest Cinnamon, or Wormwood water, then set it on a Chafing-dish of coals, and cover it close, and when it is dry, wet it again, which do so often, until the sent of the hot water be strong in it, and lay it very hot to the Stomach,

H and

and renew it once or twice in a week.

For the Winde in the Veins.

Take powder of Liquorish, Caroway-seed and Sugarcandy beaten small, of each an equal quantity to your taste, to which put Rhubarb in powder, a third part or more, with as much Cream of Tartar pulverised; put it in a box, and keep it in your pocket, and eat as much of it as will lie on a six pence, twice or thrice in a day for a week together, This will gently purge you, cool the blood, and expel the Winde out of the Veins. This hath holpen those that have not been able to go.

An excellent Sear-cloth for a Bruise, Strain or Wound.

Take one pint of Oyl Olive, red Lead eight ounces, Virgins Wax four ounces, Oyntment of Populeon four ounces, the Oyls of Roses and Cammomil, of each one ounce, set the Oy on the fire, then melt the Wax in it then put in the Populeon and Oyls, an
wh

when all are molten, put in the red lead, stir them well together, and let it boil till it be black, then dip in your clothes, and apply them to the places ill-affected.

Mr. Lumléys *Chyrurgeon. His Pippin drink for a Consumption.*

Take the thick paring of six Pippins, boil them in three pints of Spring-water to a quart, then sweeten it with Sugar-candy, whereof drink the quantity of a Wine glass when you go to bed. In a Feaver it is very good with a little Syrup of Lemons.

An approved Medicine for the Spleen.

Drink for three mornings together pure Whey, as it comes naturally from the Curd: the first morning two pints, the second morning three pints, the third morning four pints. The best exercise after it is gentle riding.

A rare Balsam.

Take Venice Turpentine one pound,

wash it four times with fair water, and as many times in Damask Rose-water, till it be as white as snow, then take an earthen pot of a Galon, make a hole in the bottom of it, which stop with a cork and a rag, and tie a string about the cork, into which pot put five pints of pure Oyl Olive, and three pints of Spring-water, boil this half a quarter of an hour, then melt eight ounces of yellow Wax in a skillet, which put to the Turpentine in the pot, take it off the fire, and stir them together with a spoon, till they be well mingled, then pluck the cork out of the earthen pot, and let out all the Water in a platter, and the Oyl and the Turpentine into the Wax in a large bason, and set them over the fire stirring them well, then pour all out into a large earthen pan, and when it is through cold, melt it again on the fire, so that it will slip out, then pour out the water in the bottom, and melt it again on the fire, stirring all well together, and so put it up into Galli-pots for your use, and you have a most excellent Balsam made by decoction, whose effects follow.

The Vertues of it.

1. It is good for any inward wound squirted warm into it, and outwardly to it on fine Lint, and anointing the place. It also preserveth the wound from inflamation and putrefaction.

2. It heals any bruise or cut being first anointed therewith, and then a peice of lint dipped in it, and laid to the place.

3. It cures all burnings and scaldings.

4. It helps the Head-ach, anointing the Nostrils and Temples therewith.

5. It expelleth the winde Cholck, or stitch in the side, being anointed and applied four mornings with warm cloths, and every morning bathing it before the fire a quarter of an hour.

6. It helps a Surfet, taking one ounce thereof in warm Sack.

7. It preserveth from the Plague, onely by anointing the Lip and Nostrils therewith before the party goeth abroad in the morning.

8. It is good against Cancers and Worms, applied as before for a cut.

9. It helps digestion and keepeth

from Vermin, if the Navel or Stomach be anointed therewith, before the party goeth to bed.

The Operator that made it, healed himself being sorely scalded.

To cure the Rickets in Children. Approved.

Take a quart of new Milk, put into it one handful of Sanicle, boil it half away, and give it to the Patient childe to drink in the morning for a breakfast, and let it not eat any thing for an hour or two after it: and at night take a quart of Milk, and one handful of red Mints, boil it half away as before, and let the Childe eat it last at night. This continue for a moneth, or longer, as occasion is. This quantity of Milk so made will serve for twice.

An Unguent to anoint the Ricketted Childes Breast.

Take fresh Butter, Sanicle, red Mints, of each one pound, stamp the Hearbs very small, then mix it with the Butter to a perfect Unguent, and therewith anoint the childes Breast every morning

ing and evening before the fire, you must anoint it from arm to arm, that it may open the breast, and also anoint the gullet bones, that they may open, for in this disease they will seem to close.

To anoint the Ricketted Childes Limbs, and to recover it in a short time, though the Childe be so lame, as to go upon Crutches.

Take a peck of Garden Snails, and bruise them, put them into a course Canvas bag, and hang it up, and set a dish under to receive the liquor that droppeth from them, wherewith anoint the Childe in every Joynt which you perceive to be weak before the fire every morning and evening. This I have known made a Childe that was extream weak to go alone, using it onely a weeks time.

For an Ague, a Plaister.

Take strong leaf Tobacco six drams, Currans a small handful, and as much Bores grease as will make it into a salve, by beating and stamping together in a mortar,

Mortar of stone; when it is beaten to a salve, take two pieces of sheeps leather, and spread the salve an inch thick on both of them; and lay them upon the veins of both wrists twenty four hours before the fit cometh. This will cure either a quartane or tertian Ague.

A dainty cooling drink for a hot Feaver.

Take French Barley one ounce, boil it first in a quart of fair water a good while, then shift it, and boil it in another quart of water a good while, shift it again, and boil it in a pottle of running Spring water to a quart, then take two ounces of sweet Almonds, lay them to soak all night, then stamp and strain them into the last Barley-water; put to it four spoonfuls of Damask Rose-water, the juyce of one Lemon, and with Sugar sweeten it to your taste, drink of this often in the night, or when you are dry or hot.

To clear the Stomach, and comfort it.

Take a pint of Sherry Sack, put in it two ounces of Jean Treacle, and four

four ounces of white Sugarcandy, boil them into a Syrup with a soft fire, and take one spoonful in the morning fasting.

A Plaister for the same.

Take a red Rose Cake, and toast the upper side of it at the fire, stick it thick full of Cloves, and dip it in a little quantity of *Aqua vitæ* and white Wine Vinegar warmed very hot in a Chafing-dish of coals, lay it to the Stomach as hot as can be suffered, and binde it fast on all night.

For a Rupture.

Take a sheet of Cap Paper, wet it in water, and fold it so wet, and lay it upon the Rupture, the party lying upon his back, but close up the Rupture first with your fingers, and so binde it down until it be dry, and then it will hold and grow with the flesh, you may wear a Truss upon it if you will.

To procure speedy Deliverance to a woman in Labour with Childe.

Take a pint of Ale, and boil it, and put to it a Womans Milk to make a Posset of it, and let the VVoman in Travel drink it; this hath procured easie and speedy Deliverance to divers women in Childe-birth.

To cure a great Flux, or Looseness of the Belly.

Take a hard Egg, and peel off the shell, and put the smaller end of it hot to the Fundament or Arse-hole, and when that is cold, take another such hot, fresh, hard and peeled Egg, and apply it as aforesaid.

For to strengthen weak Eyes Mr. Stepkins.

Take one pint of red Rose-water, Sugarcandy one ounce, Lapis Tutia two drams, both finely pulverised, put them into the Rose-water, and stir them well together, and after it hath stood twenty four hours, wet a bit of new clean spung spunge in the said water, and wash the sore eyes therewith lying backward, and when the water is almost spent, put into the glass more red Rose-water.

A rare Oyl, or Saint Johns-wort.

Take a quart of Oyl Olive, one pint of white VVine, two handfuls of Saint Johns-wort stripped seeds and all, bruise them, and put them into the Oyl, and put to it Oyl of Turpentine two ounces; put all into a great double glass close stopped, and set in the Sun ten dayes; then put the glass, with all that is in it, into a Kettle of water, with some hay or straw in the bottom, and let the water boil gently for ten or twelve hours, then strain the Hearbs from the Oyl, into which Oyl put as much fresh Saint Johns-wort and seeds bruised, and let it stand ten dayes more in the Sun: this Oyl will be then of a deep red colour, and will last seven years; it is good to heal any wound, the venemous bitings of Dogs or Serpents, and for Sprains.

A Glyster for a hot Feaver.

Take one handful of French Barley, boil it a while in water till it be red, then pour off the water, and put the Barley into a quart of running water, with Mallow and Strawberry leaves of each one handful, a few dried Cammomil flowers, and a spoonful of Anniseeds bruised, then boil it half away, and strain it out, put to the liquor a Sawcer of Oyl Olive, and four ounces of brown Sugar, with four spoonfuls of Syrup of Violets, use it something more then lukewarm.

An excellent Drink to keep ones Mouth moist.

Take of Rosemary, Cinquefoil, and a stick of Liquorish bruised, seethe them in a quart of fair water till half be consumed, then strain it from the hearbs, and put in Sugarcandy, and let it seethe a while again, and then take it off the fire, and let the Patient drink thereof cold or Luke-warm.

To stay Vomiting.

Seethe a good quantity of Cloves in Ale very well, that it may be strong of the Cloves, then sweeten it with Sugar, and drink it warm.

An excellent Receipt for Swounding, and bringing quickly to Life.

Take of the common round black Pepper, and bruise it a little, and take half a sheet of white paper, and fold it up together, and between every fold strew some of the same, and burn the one end thereof in the fire, and hold it to the Nostrils, it is very good

Against Fainting.

Take of Amber and scrape it, and put it in a spoonful of hot broth, and take it in the morning fasting, or at other time when you finde your self faint, and fast an hour after.

Dr.

Dr. Lukeners *Medicine to strengthen the Back.*

Take a pottle of fair water, and a Cock Chicken, then take three French Crowns weight of Sassafras, as much of China wood, one dram of Orange roots, one dram of Marsh Mallow roots, scrape and cut all these in small pieces, and put them in a close Pipkin, and paste it fast, that no air come out; and let it stand twenty four hours upon the fire and stew, but never boil; then open the Pipkin, and put in one French Crowns weight of Fennil-seed, and red Rose leaves, Borage, Bugloss, and Rosemary flowers, of each a small quantity, of Prunes and Raisins of the Sun each a handful, the bottom of a Manchet, boil all these together very well, till it come to a pretty thick broth, then strain it, and let the Patient take of this a reasonable draught at eight in the morning, and at four in the afternoon three dayes together.

To hold Urine.

Take the Claws of a Goat, and burn them to powder, and let the sick use hereof in their pottage a spoonful at once, it will help them.

To stay Looseness.

Take Sage, and dry it on the fire between two dishes, and then put it in a linnen bag, and sit upon it as hot as you can suffer it, and continue it till you finde ease.

A singular Medicine that the Points of the Small Pocks be not seen.

Take a fat piece of Beef being throughly powdered, and boil it a great while, then take a good quantity of the fattest broth, and strain it, and put thereto a quantity of red Rose-water, and beat them well together a good while, and when the Pocks begin to itch, anoint two or three times a day herewith till they be clean gone, and when the party is throughly well, let them

them take the broath of lean powdered Beef, and mingle it with white Wine, and so let them wash their Face therewith, and it shall bring it to smoothness, and colour, as it was before; in any wise keep not the throat nor face too hot.

To dry up the Small Pocks.

Take half a pint of new Cream, and as much Saffron as will make it of a deep Saffron colour, and boil together half a quarter of an hour, and keep it in a glass, and when the Pocks begin to wheal, warm some of the Oyntment in a Sawcer, and anoint them with a feather twice a day till they be dried up.

Dr. Eaglestones Cure for the Small Pocks or Measles.

Take a quart of Ale or Beer, and seethe it in a skillet, and put thereto a good handful of Fennil, and six or seven Figs scraped, and cut in pieces, two good spoonfuls of Anniseeds and a little Saffron, put all these to the drink, and let them seethe together till the liquor be more then half consumed, and in the

see:

seething scum it clean, and strain it into a bason, and when it is cold, make a Posset of the same drink, and use to drink this often warm, and it will cause the disease to come forth.

A most excellent Medicine that the Small Pocks be not seen in the Face.

When the smallest Pocks are cleanly come forth, and that they begin to dry, take Sperma Ceti, and warm it in a Sawcer, and with a feather anoint all the places oftentimes in the day, as often as it drieth up, that no points of the Pocks or any other spot shall be seen.

To keep the Small Pocks out of the Throat.

Take a little Saffron, and dry it by the fire, beat it into powder, and so boil it with a little Milk, and drink thereof morning and evening, and it is excellent both to keep them out of the Throat, and to bring them kindely out, that they be not within the body to endanger them.

An Oyntment for the Small Pocks when they begin to change at top, and to prevent Holes. Proved.

Take a piece of fat rusty Bacon, and scrape away the outside very pure, then tie it up to a spit, and set a pewter bason with fair water underneath the same, and let the Bacon drop therein, and when the fat of it is dropped away, then with a spoon beat that and the water together a quarter of an hour, then let it stand till it be throughly cold, then put the water out, and put the Lard into another dish of fair water; so doing for four times, then after in like sort three times, with red Rose-water, then putting the water from it, being throughly, put it up in a Galli-pot; when you will use it melt it, and with a Feather anoint the Face day and night, once in a quarter of an hour, till the Scabs be clean off, and afterwards as long as there remaineth any scurfe.

To take the Small Pocks out of the Eyes.

Take a blade or two of the biggest Saffron, and put that and Womans milk together, and so let it lie half an hour, and then with a feather anoint every quarter of an hour the out and inner sides of the Eye-lids round about as long as it is thought any Pox will come out; this will preserve the Eyes from all danger: use the like to the Nostrils, that the breath be not stopped.

An excellent one for the Small Pocks when they have appeared, and the party taken Cold. Proved.

Take a good handful of Cammomil, and not the flowers but the leaves, then seethe the same, and make Posset drink thereof, and let it taste very strong of the cammomil, but take the curd away, then drink a good draught thereof very hot four or five times, or as often as need requireth, until the Pocks appear again; this is also very excellent to stay any looseness in the body; if it should be too bitter, you may put a little sugar in it.

A Medicine to drive out the Small Pocks.

Take of distilled Taragon water eight spoonfuls, and put thereto six grains of Bezar or Unicorns horn, or for want of those two, put so much Saffron, but the other is the better: let it be warm, double the portion as you see cause, taking nothing an hour before, nor an hour after.

Another of the same, and to preserve from being infected.

Take a Quart of new Milk, put thereto half a penniworth of English Saffron powdered, boil it till it be strong and yellow, give thereof a good draught warm in the morning fasting; take it every nine dayes three mornings together, mixed with Ivory and Harts-horn, of each a small spoonful. Use it as long as you fear infection.

Dr. Stevens for the Gout: Proved.

Take two pound of Virgins Wax,

of Bores greafe half an ounce, of Sheeps fuet two ounces, of Neats-foot Oyl two ounces, of Plantane and Rofe-water each two drams, of Spike-water one dram, of Dragon-water half an ounce, as much of Borage-water, and Dr. *Stevens* water, two Nutmegs, twelve Cloves, and fome Mace of the belt, beat them fmall together, and put them into a pot, and boil it over a foft fire, until it become a Salve; then chafe the place where the party is grieved as hot as he may fuffer, and then fpread it on a fine linnen cloth, and lay it upon the place fix or eight dayes.

The Countefs of Mounteagles *excellent Medicine for the Cramp. Proved.*

Take a handful of the Hearb called Perriwinkle, fome of it beareth a blew flower, and fome white, and alfo take a good handful of Rofemary tops, put them into a Pewter-difh, and fet them upon coals, dry them and turn them very often, and when they are very hot, lay them upon the place that is fo taken with the Cramp, and binde a cloth upon them, when you go to bed, and

and this will help you, take it in the morning, and lay fresh at night.

A Posset-drink for one that is Heart sick to remove it thence, though it be the Plague.

Take Ale and make Posset-drink thereof, and clarifie it, then take Pimpernel, and seethe in it till it be strong of it, and drink often thereof.

Remedies against the Falling-sickness.

Take Powder of Harts-horn, drink it with Wine, it helpeth that disease: so do Ravens Eggs taken with the juyce of Wilde Rue, and the juyce of Misletoe.

To avoid Phleagm.

Take clarified Posset-drink, and put thereto sweet Butter, the yolk of an Egg, and a little small Ginger, Hysop, red Mints and Sugar, let these seethe all together; and drink thereof first and last as warm as you can suffer it.

A very good means to stay a Looseness that happeneth in Childe bed.

First in the water you mean to use, quench a gad of Steel sundry times, then take the inward barks of the Sloe, of the Brambles, and of the young Oak, of each a like quantity, and so much as will suffice according to the liquor you intend to make; if you use three pints of water, a pretty handful of each bark will serve finely scraped; when they are well boiled, that one pint is wasted, strain your liquor, and make it into Almond Milk, with unblanched Almonds finely grown, then with well boiled Ivy thicken your Milk, and other Rice broth, and season it with Sugar and Cinnamon finely beaten, let the party forbear drink as much as may be, and eat thereof once in two or three hours, a little at once, as her stomach will serve. If she have any gripe in her Belly, I wish this to be used, which I know to be singular good for any stoppage by sudden cold in Childebed. Gather a great deal of Cammomil, and heat it well between two
Char-

Chargers upon a Chafing-dish of Coals, and when the moisture of the Hearb is somewhat spent, strew in a handful of bruised Cummin-seed, and sprinkle it now and then with a little Malmsey, and so being a little dryish, put it into a thin bag, and apply it to the belly as hot as may be suffered, and as it cooleth warm it again, till she have ease: instead of Malmsey you may use Muscadine. This hath been many times proved.

For a Knock or Bruise in the Face.

Take a piece of brown paper, and wet it in Beer, and lay it where the knock is, and as it beginneth to dry, lay on fresh a good while together.

For a Wen.

Take Stone Lime and put it into water, till it have done boiling, then take a quantity of it, and mix it with some barrel Soap, laying them both on a cloth, let it be applied to it, and it will eat away the Wen.

For

Mr. Potter *Chyrurgem. His Cure for a Man that is burſten.*

Take the roots of bake Fern, and the roots of Elecampane, of each a like quantity, waſh and pare them clean, cut them as ſmall as you can, and ſtamp them in a Mortar as fine as you can, and temper it with Oyl of Bay, and two ſpoonfuls of Oyl of Exceter, and when you have made the Salve, ſpread it upon his Cod to his Belly, and lay the Plaiſter upon the hole, and remove it every two dayes, and then uſe another ſpace of ten dayes, you muſt uſe another Salve or Plaiſter as followeth. Take a quarter of a pound of   and the white of three or four Eggs, and temper them together; and when they are well tempered, put in two ſpoonfuls of Peſ-colium; temper all theſe together, and uſe the ſame as you did the former ſalve; when you take off the Plaiſter, you muſt lay fine clothes under the bolſter of the Truſs, until you think the skin be grown.

A Medicine to deſtroy Warts.

Take Radiſh root, and ſhred it thin,

I   and

and put it in a pewter dish, and cast salt upon it, and cover it with another dish, and shake the slices up and down, and then take a piece thereof, and rub the Warts therewith, then throw away that, and use another so three or four times in a day.

To take away Corns.

Take Hogs Grease that is not tried, and beat it with a Pestle, and spread it upon a piece of white Cotten on the rugged side, and binde it on the Corns, dressing it once or twice a day, and it will wear them away.

To take away Freckles or Morphew.

Take four spoonfuls of May dew, and one spoonful of the Oyl of Tartar, mingle them together, and wash the places where the Freckles be, and let it dry of it self, it will clear the skin, and take away all foul spots.

The Lady Nevil for a sore breast, by cold or festring of Milk.

Take of Beans and Linseed, of each one little handful, dry them and beat them to powder, then take a quantity of Milk, and the Yolk of two new laid Eggs, and boil them together, then put in the powder of Beans and Linseed, and boil it to a Poultess, and lay it to the breast as hot as may be endured, and it will both draw and heal it; dress it twice in a day.

Dr. Soper his Water for a sore Eye, or any Defect or Decay in the Sight.

Take of red, or rather of white Rose-water half a pint, Lapis Celaminaris half an ounce, Lapis Lucius as much, beat them both to powder, and finely searse them, the dropping of Dale, Rhenish Wine half a pinte, Honey half a spoonful, mix whole Cloves, Plantain-water half a quarter of a pint, of the Drugs of Aloes as much as a Walnut beaten to powder, and finely searsed, shake them very well together half an hour

hour or more, then let them stand twenty four hours before you begin to use it, stop it close, and it will be good a year, when you use it, you must put in a drop with a quil into the corner of the eye, and let the party lean back a quarter of an hour; use it morning and evening.

To take a white skin from the Eye that came by some blow, though a quarter of a year since.

Take the gall of a white Cock Chicken, and a drop or two of Life Honey, mingle them together in a Sawcer on a few Embers, and drop it three or four times a day into the Eye.

For breaking out of yong Childrens Heads.

Take Butter and Salt, and fry it together till it be black, and when it is cold, anoint their head. Or else take pure Sallat Oyl and Vinegar, and beat them together, anoint the place morning an evening till it be whole. Whey mad with Agrimony and Scabious, an Wormwood, is excellent to clear th blood.

An excellent Medicine for a Scald, or Burn newly done.

Take Horse-dung newly made, or as new as you can get, and strain it through a thin old cloth, and therewith anoint the place two or three times a day, and every time dip the cloth in the Horse-dung, so strain it, and binde it to the sore all Day and Night, it will cure you.

The Countess of Arundels *Drink for the Scurvey.*

Take of Fumitory and Scurvy-grass, that which grows by the Sea side, of each twelve little handfuls, of Brook-lime three little handfuls, of Water-Cresses six little handfuls, wash and dry them very clean, and stamp them, and hang them in three galons of strong Beer or Ale, when it is stale, drink a good draught in the morning, fasting an hour after, another an hour before dinner, and another half an hour before you go to bed, the more exercise you use after it the better, it is needful to

be

be well purged, before you take this drink or any other, use it three weeks or a moneth together; if you cannot have green Fumitory, use dry.

Paracelsus *his Plaister called* Emplastrum Fodicatonum Paracelsi, *good for many Diseases herein mentioned, Translated out of Latine into English.*

Take of the four Gums, that is to say, Galbanum, Opoponax, of each one dram, Ammoniacum, and Bedellium, of each two drams, let them be beaten very small, and put them in an earthen pot leaded or glazed, pouring upon the same very good Vinegar of Wine, and let them so remain a day and night, then boil them in the same Vinegar upon a great fire, that the Gums may melt, and when they be throughly melted, pour out the same hot into a bag, wring or press the same, that they may be well cleansed from the dregs, which dregs must be cast away, take the said Liquor so strained out, and let it boil till the Vinegar be wasted, and utterly evaporated; in the boiling you must continually
stir

stir it without ceasing, lest the Gums be burned, keep this very clean and covered, that nothing fall into it, then take Oyl Olive two pound, new Wax half a pound, and let them be put into an earthen pot, well leaded or glazed of a sufficient bigness, set the same on a fire of coals, and let them melt at leisure; at the length put into it a pound and half of Lithargie beaten into very fine powder, stirring it continually with a stick or spatula by little and little, until it be throughly mixt together, and the matter be a tawny colour; afterwards take the aforesaid Gums that were first boiled, and put the quantity of a Nut into the said matter; and so by little and little at several times, put into it such like quantity of the Gums at each time, till the Gums be all put in, and mixt well with the other things, and melted. And you must take heed withal, lest the matter be overmuch heated, and boil over and run into the fire, for it is very hot of it self, afterwards put in the things following into it, of the two kindes of Aristolichia rotunda, Calaminaris, Myrrhe and Frankincense, of each one dram, beat them into fine powder,

der, that are to be made into powder, and put them into the said matter, and pour on it one dram of Oyl of Bays, and put therein lastly four drams of white Turpentine, boil them and stir them about continually with careful diligence, and when you will know whether it be sufficiently sodden, put a little thereof into cold water, and if it be not so soft that it cleave to your fingers, it is well, otherwise it must boil longer, then take it from the fire, and pour it into a bason full of water, and when it is well cooled, that you may handle it, anoint your hand with Oyl of Cammomil or Roses, and knead it well three or four hours, and so lay it up in a cleansed vessel, it will last above fifty years, and be then as good as at the first day it was made.

The Vertues of the Emplaister out of Paracelsus.

It is good for old or new Sores, it drieth, cleanseth, and breedeth good flesh, it confirmeth and comforteth, it healeth more in a week, then any other in a moneth, it will not suffer any Sore to putrefie or corrupt, or any dead or evil flesh to grow, for sinnews cut, bruised or pricked with a Thorn or otherwise, it is most excellent; it draweth out of Wounds Iron, Wood or Lead, and other the biting of venemous Beasts; it causeth all kinde of Imposthumes or Biles to ripen, if it be laid thereon, and it is most excellent against the Canker and Fistula, the Shingles or Saint Anthonies fire; and also a soveraign and speedy help against all paines, to asswage all aches, and for all kinde of wounds; also I *Thomas Potter* have found often experience, it is singular and special help for bones out of joynt, by laying one or two plaisters, or three at the most: I have healed in fourteen dayes Arms out of joynt, so that those parties have said they have had no pain nor weakness after. Also for thrusts you must not tent them, unless they matter before you come to them, but onely lay of this over it, and two plaisters is commonly sufficient to heal it, or any other sore or swelling, but if dead flesh be in a sore before this Plaister be laid on, it will not destroy it, but it must be pluckt out, but if it finde none, it will suffer none to breed. When you lay up this Plaister, put it in oyled paper or

oyled

Oyled leather, or both, it will keep it the better for over much drying, and you must lay it out of the Sun and Winde.

For the biting of a mad Dog, or stinging of an Adder.

Take a handful or more of Hazle-Nuts, a quarter as much of Rue, with a Clove of Garlick, stamp all these together, then take the juyce, and put a little Treacle to it, and if it be a man that is stung or bitten, give it him to drink in Beer, or Wine, or Ale; but if a dog, give it in Milk; then take that from whence the juyce came, and binde it to the place which was bit or stung.

For the biting of a Snake.

Stamp Garlick, and lay it to the place that is bitten.

Dr. Lukeners, *For one stung with Waspe.*

Make a little Plaister of Treacle, and lay it upon the place that is so stung, and it will help it.

Physical and Chyrurgical Receipts. 155

An Oyntment for a great or hard Belly, by Ague, Worms, or Spleen.

Take the finest common Wormwood, Garden Tanfey, Featherfew, Lavender, Cotten, Southern-wood, Unfet Leeks blades, and all Pearch Leaves, Herbgrace, of each one little handful, wash them and dry them; then take a good pound of Barrows greafe, and stamp all in a wooden dish, then set them eight or nine dayes in a Sellar, or low place till they have a Hoar all over them; then break them all together, and put them in an earthen pot, and set them on a soft fire, and let them boil a good hour, then strain them through a clean cloth into a Gallipot or Glafs, and so keep it for a precious Oyntment; it will last a year well; when you ufe it, you must warm it, and anoint the belly of the Patient morning and evening. Proved by Miftrefs *Joyce*, Widow.

The old Lady of Oxfords Oyl of Excester which is good for all maner of cold Gouts, Sciatica, and all manner of Aches in the Flesh and Bones, and also for Bruises. Proved.

Take one pound of Cowslip-flowers, picked out of their cases, gathered in *April* on a fair day when the Dew is gone, and souse them in Oyl Olive, so much as will cover them, let them lie in it till *June* in a glass, then take Calamint, Hearb John, Sage, Agrimony, Southern-wood, Pellitory of Spain, Rosemary, Wormwood, Penniroyal, Lavender, Cammomil, Hirse, Lawrel leaves, flower of Lillies, Pellitory and Featherfew, the tenderness of the Ivy and Broom-flowers, of each one little handful; stamp them all together well, and then infuse them in White Wine, so that they may be covered all over therein, so let them remain fourteen hours or fifteen, then put them in Oyl Olive, so that the liquor may near swim, so boil it together upon a soft fire, and stir it well till the rawness and wetness of the Oyl be gone, then strain it through

a

a Canvas cloth into a pewter dish, or glass, for earth or wood will not hold it, and use it for a singular good Oyntment, and above all other approved, if there be any pieces in the pan which the said Oyl is boiled in, it wil run out, after the hearbs are once hot, it must be continually stirred on a very little fire, no more then any Egg will abide without breaking.

To make a Sear-cloth against Swellings and Aches. Approved.

Take Bloom-flowers two little handfuls, red Bramble leaves one little handful, this Bramble beareth but three leaves together, and groweth low on the ground, take it off on the middle leaf, a piece of unwashed Butter, and pound the Hearbs aforesaid with two or three Cloves, and then boil them in Butter, and strain it, and take a peice thereof, with a little piece of Wax, and being melted together, make a Sear-cloth with it. Also take Oyl of Broom, Bramble and Butter, and temper it with a little Aqua vitæ; it is good against Aches, to be used and rubbed on the aches in the morning, but not at night.

The

The Lady Leonards green Oyntment.

Take red Sage leaves, and Rue of each one pound, the youngest Bay leaves and Wormwood, of each half a pound, gather these in the heat of the day, pick them, wash them not, cut them small, and beat them long in a fair Mortar, then take half a pound of Sheeps Suet hot from the Sheep, mince it small and put it to the hearbs, beat it together till it is all of one colour, then put all into a clean bowl, put to it a pottle of the best Oyl Olive, work all these well until all become a like soft, then put it into an earthen pot well stopt for eight dayes; then with a soft fire seethe it in a fair pan, put to it four drams of Oyl of Spike, when it is half sodden; being sodden, strain it through a clean Canvas into clean Gallipots stopt close with Parchment and double Sheeps leather, anoint the place grieved therewith, rubbing it every day before you leave it, if you put a clean warm cloth after you have anointed the place thereon it is better: this is made onely in *May*, and will last many years being close stopt, and cool kept.

The Lady Smith's Remedy to bring a young Childe when it is born.

Take a little Coventry Blew Thred, burn it, and hold it to the Childes Nose, that the smoak may go up.

To bring away the After burthen although a day or two after the Delivery.

Take Rie, and crede it as you do Wheat for Furmity, and make a Caudle of it, so let her drink a good draught once or twice. This is proved.

For one bound in body, though a Woman with Childe.

Take a pinte of White Wine, a quarter of a pint of Damask Rose-water, twenty Damask Prunes, forty Raisins of the Sun stoned, a little whole Mace, and a few Anniseeds tied in a cloth; let all these boil leasurely together, and put thereto either Sugarcandy or fine Sugar, and when it is boiled to a Syrup take out a little of it, and strain it through a fine cloth with a little Manna, and put into the Syrup; and let it simper together

ther a good while, then put it into a glass, it will keep good a good while, as half a year, and when you have occasion to use it, you must take one of the said Prunes, and two or three Raisins, and eat them in the morning fasting, and take a spoonful also of the said Syrup fasting two or three hours after the same.

Dr. Atkinsons *Glister for Winde*

Take Cammomil, Mallows, Violet leaves, Bert leaves, Bean and French Barley one little handful, of Fennel-seed and Anniseed each two spoonfuls; boil all these together with a Rack of Mutton, till the flesh be very tender; then take a pint of the fattest liquor strained and put into it two drams of the Oyl of Rue, or Oyl of Cammomil, and for want thereof a little dish Butter melted, two drams of course Sugar, and one or two yolks of Eggs

To bring away a dead child, or afterburden.

Take Saffron, Mace and Cinnamon, beat them to powder, and searce them; and

and take of the powder a just quantity, give as much as will lie upon the point of a knife in Ale, Beer, or one spoonful of what they best like.

A gentle Purge which taketh away a Tertian Ague, being given the fourth Fit. Proved.

Take a dram of Rhubarb, and infuse it in Succory-water six spoonfuls, three hours together on a very gentle fire, then strain it, and put it in half a dram of Syrup of Rhubarb, three spoonfuls of Syrup of Roses, and a spoonful of Cinnamon-water, take this fasting after the fourth fit when they are not sick; if this be too weak to purge a strong body, add thereunto two or three drams of the leaves of Sena, with a few Fennil-seed to quicken it more, if it be alwayes made with this addition, it is the better.

The Lady Gorings Water for an Ague, Sickness, or foulness in the Stomach, and to purge the Blood.

Take the Dung of a Stone-horse that is kept in the stable, when it is new made, mingle it well with Beer and a little
Ginger,

Ginger, and a good quantity of Treacle, and diſtil it in an ordinary ſtill; give of this a pretty draught to drink.

The Lady Gorings Remedy for a Burn or Scald.

Take Hogs Fat or Seam made of it, melt it, but let it not boil, put into it the white of a new laid Egg or two well beaten, and ſtir it continually on Embers, till it be like an Oyntment; keep it for your uſe, anointing the ſore twice a day with it.

The Lady Gorings Remedy for a ſharp Urine.

Boil running-water with Liquoriſh till it be ſomething ſtrong of it, boil alſo in it a Pippin or two, when it is boiled, put in alſo ſome brown Sugarcandy, drink of it every morning faſting a pretty draught.

For Deafneſs. Proved.

Take Linſeed Oyl and *Aqua vitæ*, ſhake them together in a glaſs bottle, and ſet it in the Sun a moneth or five weeks, ſhake

...ake it well every day, and when you ...e it, put a little into the ear, and stop it ...ith a little black Wool.

An Approved Receipt to stop Bleeding at the Nose, Wound or Cut in man or beast.

Take the flax of a Hare, the Moss of ...n Ash tree, and powder of Bolearmo-...ck, chop them together, and wet them ...little with fair water, and put it into ...he Nostril that bleeds, and stir it not ...twenty four hours; if it be of a cut or ...ound, look first if there be not little ...ieces of loose flesh or skin that hangs, ...there be, clip it away, or else the ...lood will not stay, then lay the aforesaid ...edicine to it, and stir it not in twenty ...ur hours.

The Lady Nevils Remedy for the Stone.

Take the hearb Aurea, or Gold Wire, ...ry it and keep it all the year, and every ...ull of the Moon take a spoonful of ...he powder in six spoonfuls of Milk, ...nd water, and one of white Wine, or ...ou may take it in Plantain-water, or ...ervin-water, or any that is good for the

the Stone, it is also good to take it in the fit.

The Lady Mildmayes Drink for Cough or Cold.

Take of Liquorish scraped and sliced, of Anniseeds rubbed and bruised, of Raisins of the Sun stoned, of Figs sliced, of Hysop tops, of each one little handful, and a great handful of Coltsfoot; boil all these in a galon of running water, until two or three parts be consumed, then strain it, and stir it in three or four good spoonfuls of Honey, take this in the morning fasting, at four a clock in the afternoon, and when you go to bed four spoonfuls at a time warm.

Mrs. Chaunce, her Receipt for the Spleen, and Melancholy, the Preparative.

Take of the roots of Parsley, Fennil, Bruscus, Sparagus, of each four ounces, the seeds of Fennil, Annise and Caraway, of each a dram and half, of the bark of Capers and Tamarisk, of each an ounce and half, of the leaves of Mugwort, Borage, Buglofs, of each one little handful,

of

Cetrach and Dictamum each one little handful, boil all these things in three pints of Conduit-water, till half thereof be consumed, then strain it, and put to it Syrup of Harts-tongue, and Syrup of Succory, and Rhubarb in powder, or sliced each four ounces, then let it stand all night, and the next day clarifie it, and after put to it the spices of Letificans Galeni, and Diamuscum Dulce, each two scruples, take of this in the morning fasting six ounces, and as much an hour before supper, take it thus two dayes together, then take the Purge following.

Mrs. Chaunce *her Purge.*

Take of Sena three drams, of Epithimum and Polypody of the Oak each two drams, of Fennil, Annise, and Caraway seeds, each a dram and a half, Cardus seed two scruples, boil them all in a sufficient quantity of Conduit-water, until it come to three ounces, then put to it of Rhubarb a dram and a half, infused in Succory water, of the Syrup of Augustanus, and Syrup of Harts-tongue each one ounce, to make a Potion

tion, and take it three times, every third day take one of these, and take at night when you go to bed, of Diascordium two scruples, of Alkerms dissolved in Borage-water one dram.

Mr. Powel for the Stone and Cholick.

Take the quantity of half an Hazle-nut kernel and Mithridate, and so much black Sope, and mix them together, and take a broad Onion, and cut off the top, and make it somewhat hollow, and put the black Sope and Mithridate in it, and cover it with the piece you cut off, wrap it it in Paper, and roast it in Embers until it be very soft; then put it between two linnen clothes warm, and lay to the Navil, and pin the clothes upon the back, so use it till you finde ease.

Mr. Rowland Hauglitons Receipt for the cure of the Stone.

Take Arsemart, otherwise called red Shank, and distill it, and take it in the Evening when you are warm in bed, to the quantity of half a pint, and the like in the morning a little before you rise,

Physical and Chyrurgical Receipts.   167

...se, about some four times, then take ...arberries, and take the outside Rinde of ...em, and beat them into very fine pow-...er, and take every morning and even-...g, and drink either a draught of the said ...Water, or small Beer after it: continue ...is, and it will cure you.

For an Ague congealed, or fallen into a Womans Breast.

Take a quantity of stone Honey, and ...he rustiest Bacon you can get, Smallage, ...lexander, red Cole, Marigolds with ...lack seeds of Groundsel, Plantane, and ...age, of each a quantity; put all these in ... mortar and stamp them as small as you ...an, then lay the Salve upon a piece of ...hite Leather, and to the place where ...ou would have the Breast break, the ...laister must be spread upon the rough ...de of the Leather.

An approved Medicine by the Lady Bray for the Ague falling into any part of the Body.

Take of Parsley one little handfull, ...mallage and Hemlock of each as much, ...hop them small, then stamp them and
put

put thereto a quantity of Barrows grease, and stamp them all together, then boil them a good space, stirring it continually until it wax green, then strain it, and when you use thereof, take some in a Saweer, and anoint the place with a feather against the fire.

The Lady Arundels especial Remedy for the Stone, Back, or Stomach, or to make a Woman Conceive.

Take the roots of Sea-holly (it groweth by the Sea side, like little trees, of half a yard long, some name them Eringoes) and make it in Syrup, and eat of it in the morning fasting, and at four a clock in the afternoon, and before you take it, take some gentle Pills, but once in the beginning.

The Lady Dacres Medicine proved, for the Stone and Stanguary.

Take black Bramble-berries when they be red, Ivie-berries, the inner pith of Ashen Keys, Eglantine-berries, the Nut Keys, the roots of Filipendula, of all these a little, Acrons and the stones of of Sloes of each a like quantity, but not so much of either of these as half of any of the other, dry all these in platters in in Oven, till they will be beaten to powder, then take Cromel-seed, Anniseed, Saxifrage, Alexanders, Parsley, Corianders, Fennil-seeds, the seeds of each of these the like quantity of the first, and dried in like sort, then beat all together in the like sort to fine powder, then take Liquorish fair scraped the best you can get, as much in quantity as all these, and beat it fine, and mingle it with the powder, and keep it close from the winde, and so use it morning and evening with Posset Ale, with Time of the Mount boiled in it, make your Posset drink with white Wine, or other drink, and when you eat any pottage or other broth, put some of the powder in it if you be sore pained, and if you have any Stone, it will come away in shiver, and if it do so when you drink, your water is clear, take this drink following, and it will leave no corruption or uncleanness in the bladder.

The Drink.

Take Rosemary and Wilde Time, and seethe them in running water with as much Sugar as will make it sweet, boil it from a quart to a pint, use the quantity of the Hearbs to your discretion, so that it may savour of them well, and use it nine mornings, six or seven spoonfuls at a time.

Mr. Eldertons *Medicine for the extremity of the Chollick and Stone.*

Take Ashen Keys, and dry them in an Oven, take out the Kernels from the Husks, beat them into powder, and searse them fine, and keep it; then take Eglantine berries, dry and beat them as the other, then take of them with a feather, then searse it as above, take Houseleek, dry and searse it as the other, take a little quantity of the three powders, and put them together, take Anniseeds, and Liquorish of each a little quantity, dry them severally and powder them, being fine searsed, put them with the other three powders, a little quantity

of

of both, and take a spoonful of these powders or less, and mingle all together, and put into it three or four spoonfuls of white Wine or Ale, and drink it in the morning, fasting one hour after it; thus drink it once in six dayes, or else when you are grieved; and you shall never finde pain of the Cholick nor Stone. The seed of great Nettles must be beaten to powder, and mixt with them, and it will be better.

For a Pin or Web in the Eye far gone.

Take the Marrow of a Goose-wing, and mingle the powder of Ginger therewith, dress the eye therewith two or three times a day.

A Medicine for the Eye Aching, or Redness thereof.

Take a vial glass, and fill it full of fair running water, and put into it fine Sanguis Draconis, the quantity of a Hazle Nut, it will help the Eye.

For sore Eyes that come from hot Humors.

Take Elder leaves, and chafe between your hands, and lay it to the nape of the neck.

For the Pin and Web in the Eye, so it be taken before the sight be quite extinct.

Take a little handful of three leaved grass, that hath the sign of the Moon in it, as much roots and leaves of Dasies, and seven or eight corns of Bay-salt, beat all these together, then straine them through a cloth, and take two new laid Eggs, and beat the whites of them a good while, then let them stand a quarter of an hour, and then take off the froth clean, and take the clear of the whites, as much as the quantity of the juyce of the said hearbs, then take the quantity of two Hazle Nuts of English Honey and stir them together, then let the party be laid upright, and drop three drops with a feather into the Eye, and lie still a good while after, this must be used at the least twice a day.

For red Eyes, Pearl, Pin or Web.

Take Verjuyce that is made of Grapes, and put it morning and evening into the sore Eyes; some will put a little Salt with it.

Dr. Friers excellent Remedy for Heat and Pimples in the Face.

Take of Plantain leaves four little handfuls, and of Mallows or Tansey one little handful, of Cinquefoll half a little handful, and as much of Strawberry leaves, there must be this quantity of every sort; when they are pickt clean, then take a pottle of new Milk hot from the Cow, and put it in a still with the same hearbs until it be dropped a quart, then let it drop no more; you may keep it a whole year in a glass, when you use it wet a cloth in some of it, and wash your face at night to bed, and often in the day, the best time to still it is in *May*.

For Heat or Scurf in the Face.

Take a pint of Cream as thick as

can be scummed, then take of Cammomil one little handful, pick, wash and shred it very small, then put it into the cream, and let it boil very softly till it comes to an Oyl, never stirring it after the putting in the hearbs at first, but scum it clean when you see the Oyl come to the top, then let it boil a little faster, and then strain it through a fine linnen cloth, and then anoint the face therewith.

A very good Medicine for a Tetter.

Take red Dock roots, wash them, scrape them, and cut them into slices, and lay them in white Wine Vinegar a night or a day, and then use it to the place grieved, washing the place with the root, and the liquor many times.

To skin the rawness of a Womans Nipple.

Take a Deers foot, and take the marrow thereof, and anoint the nipple therewith.

To dry up Milk in a Womans Breast.

Take a quantity of *Aqua vitæ*, and a quan-

quantity of sweet Butter, melt and temper them together, and anoint the Breast therewith, laying a brown paper betwixt them, and so do as often as the paper drieth, till the Milk be dried up: this is also good to keep the Ague out of the Breast.

To make a woman have a Nipple that hath none, and would give suck.

Take a Wicker Bottle that hath a little mouth, and fill it full of hot water, and stop it close till the bottle be through hot, then let out the water, and set the mouth of the bottle close to the Nipple; as long as there is any heat in the bottle it will cleave fast.

To heal the Nipple of a Womans Breast.

Take a quantity of Cream, and put it into the juyce of Valerian stamped and strained, and as much of the juyce of seagreen used in like sort; boil all these together till it come to be as Butter; then take it, and put it into a box, and anoint the Nipple therewith three or four times a day, and lay a Walnut shel, or some other hollow thing over it to keep the clothes from it till it be whole, or else make a Posset Ale, of Alom and lay the curd to the Nipple warm, till the childe doth suck, and then lay on again.

A Medicine for Worms in young Children.

Take a plaister of white Leather or brown paper, and spread it with Honey, warm it a little against the fire, but first strew some of the best Aloes Succotrinæ thereon, then lay it all over the Stomach of the childe warm; the like plaister is to be laid on the childes Navil at the same time; if you have no Honey, mix the juyce of Plantain, and lay it on the leather.

Dr. Forsters *Infusion purging Choler.*

Take Damask Roses two ounces, of Rhubarb two drams and a half, of Spikenard one scruple, of Orcin one scruple, cut all small, and infuse in a quart of clarified whey all night, in the morning strain gently, and put to it one ounce of Syrup of Roses, or Syrup of Violets.

Dr.

Dr. Fosters Infusion purging Melancholy.

Take Fumitory, Epithymum, flowers or leaves of Borage and Bugloss, of each a good half handful, Polypody of the Oak one ounce, Sena half an ounce, Fennil-seed two drams, Whey three pints; infuse and boil to a quart, whereunto adde two ounces of Syrup of Roses solutive; the dose is half a pound, you may quicken a draught with a dram of Electuary of Roses.

An opening purging Julip, and cooling for Choler and hot Humors.

Take of Barley two little handfuls, of Savory with the roots, Maidenhair, Liverwort, Sorrel, each half a good handful, of roots of Grass of Fennil, each half an ounce, of the four cold seeds each two drams, boil them a sufficient quantity of Succory water unto sixteen ounces, in which infuse half an ounce of Sena Tamarindes, and Polypody of each three drams, Jalap and Hermodactils, of each two drams, Fennil-seed, Annifeed, and Liquorish, of each

each one dram, Currans bruised half an ounce, of Borage, Bugloss, and Rosemary flowers, of each one dram; infuse these warm, then boil them until five ounces of the Succory Water be consumed, then strain it, and adde the expression of four scruples of Rhubarb infused, in three ounces of Manna, and syrup of Roses one ounce, of the Christals of Tartar one dram, mingle them: the Dose is four or five ounces every morning.

Doctor Mores *Powder, or glosly prepared Drug to be taken in mornings, and after Meals, to mend Concoction, comfort the Brain, break Winde, and make sweet Breath.*

Take Liquorish cut small, Anniseed Comfits with one skin of Sugar, of each two ounces, sweet Fennil-seed Comfits with one skin of Sugar, Corianders prepared, and Carroway-seed of each one ounce, of white Ginger, Cinnamon, Calamus Aromaticus, and Nutmegs, of each one ounce cut very small, of the Lozenges of Aromaticum Rosatum, of Manus Christies, with Chymica, Oyl of Cinnamon, Cloves, and Lozenges of Diambra

ambra cut into small pieces, each half an ounce, to be taken about a spoonful at the times aforesaid.

Lucatellos *Balsam admirable for all Wounds.*

Take Venice Turpentine one pound, Oyl Olive three pints, Sack six spoonfuls, yellow Wax one pound, natural Balsam half an ounce, Oyl of Saint Johns-Wort, red Sanders powdered, of each one ounce, wash the Venice Turpentine three times in red Rose-water; then slice the Wax thin, and set it on the fire in a big Skillet, and when it is well molten, put the Turpentine to it, and stir them well together till they boil a little, take it off the fire, and let it cool till the next day, then cut it into thick slices, and pour all the water out of it, then set it on the fire again, and when it is molten, stir it well, and put it into the aforesaid Oyls, Sack, Balsam and Sanders, and stir them well together that they may incorporate, then let it boil again for a short space, take it off the fire, and stir it well for the space of two hours, that it may become thick,

thick, and when it is cold, put it up in several Gallipots, and when you use it, apply it tented into a deep and hollow wound, if it be onely a slit cut, anoint the wound with it, and binde it fast on with the cloth.

A Purge by Dr. Maysiern.

Take of the best Sena six drams, of Rhubarb two drams, Cream of Tartar half a dram, of sweet Fennil-seed as much, and a little Cinnamon; infuse all these one night in half a pint of white Wine, in the morning let it boil one walm or two, strain it, and put of the best Manna an ounce, dissolve it over the fire, then strain it again, then put to it an ounce of Sa'atine syrup of Roses; so drink it, fast two hours after from meat, and drink & sleep, and then drink nothing but thin broth.

An approved Medicine to beautifie the Face, or to take away Pimples or Heat in the Face.

Take a fair earthen Pipkin, and put into it a pottle of clean running water, and an ounce of white Mercury beaten

to

to white powder, then set it on the fire, and let it boil until one half be consumed, and keep it close covered saving when you stir it, then take the whites of six new laid egs beaten half an hour or more, and put it into the liquor, after it is taken from the fire, you must put in also the juice of Lemons being very good, and half a pint of new Milk, and a quarter of a pound of bitter Almonds blanched and beaten with half a pint of Damask Rose-water, strain all these together through a strainer, and let it stand three weeks before you use it, and I will warrant you fair, &c.

An excellent Water for the Eyes that are red or full of Rhume.

Take young Hazle Nuts when they are so soft, that you may thrust a pin through them, still them in a Rose still, Husks, Shells and all, and with the water wash your eyes.

To cure a Wound though the Patient be never so far off.

Take a quart of pure Spring water, and put it into some Roman Vitriol, and

and let it dissolve, then if you have any blood of the wound either in linnen or woollen, or silk, put the cloth so blooded in the water, and rub the cloth once a day, and if the wound be not mortal, the blood will out, if it be, it will not. Let the Patient keep his Wound clean, washing it with white Wine; when ever you wash the cloth, the party wounded shall sensibly finde ease: let the cloth be constantly in the water.

To make Oyl of Swallows.

Take Swallows as many as you can get, ten or twelve at the least, and put them quick into a Mortar, and put to them Lavender, Cotton, Spike, Cammomil, Knot-grass, Ribwort, Balm, Valerian, Rosemary tops, Woodbine tops, strings of Vines, French Mallows, the tops of Alehoof, Strawberry strings, Tutsane, Plantain, Walnut leaves, tops of young Bayes, Hysop, Violet leaves, Sage of vertue, fine Roman Wormwood, Brooklime, Smallage, Mother of Time, of each of these a handful, two of Cammomil, and two of red Roses, beat all these together, and put thereto a quart of

Neats-foot Oyl, or May Butter, stamp them all together, and beat them with one or two ounces of Cloves, and put them all together in an earthen pot, stop it very close with a piece of dough round about, so close that no air can come out; set them nine days in a cellar, and then take them out, and boil them six or eight hours on the fire, or else in a pan of water; but first open your pot, and put in half a pound of Wax, white or yellow, whether you will, and a pint of Sallet Oyl, and strain them through a Canvas cloth.

To make Lead Plaister.

Take two pound and four ounces of the best and greenest Sallet Oyl, with a pound of good red Lead, and a pound of white Lead, beat them well into dust, then take twelve Ounces of Castle-Sope, incorporate all these well together in a well glassed and great earthen pot, that the Sope may come upwards, set it on a small fire of coals the space of one hour and a half, alwayes stirring it with an iron ball, or round Pommil; then make your fire somewhat bigger until it it be the colour of Oyl, then drop a little on the board, and if it cleave neither to your finger nor the board, then it is enough; then take the clothes and make them into what breadth or size you please in Searcloth, let not your cloth be course, but of a reasonable new Holland; and when you have dipped them, then rub them with a Slick-stone, it will last two years, and the elder the better as long as it will stick it is good.

The Vertues of the Leaden Plaister.

1. If it be laid to the Stomach, it provoketh appetite, and taketh away any grief in the same.

2. If laid to the belly, it is a present remedy for the Ache.

3. If laid to the Reins of the back, it cureth and healeth the Bloody Flux, the running of the Reins, heat in the Liver, or weakness of the Back.

4. It healeth all Bruises and Swellings, it taketh away aches, it breaketh Fellons, Pushes, and other Impostumes, and healeth them.

5. It draweth out any running Humour without breaking of the skin, and being applied to the Fundament, it
healeth

healeth any disease there growing.

6. The same laid to the head is good for the Eyes.

7. The same laid to the Belly of a Woman, provoketh the Tearms, and maketh apt for Conception.

For the Stone and Gravel.

Take and dry the roots of red Nettles, make them into powder, and drink a spoonful of the powder in a draught of white Wine something warm, and it will break the Stone, though it be never so great with speed, use it every day until the Stone and Gravel be all broken and consumed. A thing of small price, and great vertue.

A drink to purge the body, being very good for them that have the Scurvey, or are inclined to it.

Take a pottle of fine running water, and a pint of Rhennish Wine for a young body, and for any elder, take a quart, set it on the fire, put into it three or four slices of Horse Radish, a great handful of Water Cresses, and a handful

ful of Brooklime, both a little bruised, slice in two or three Oranges, outsides and insides, let them boil all together better then half an hour, then have ready a greater quantity of Scurvy-grass bruised, or a pint of the Juyce of Scurvy-grass ready strained, and put into the liquor, and set over the fire again, then there will arise a curd, which being taken off, put it into the drink when it is cold, three or four Lemons more, or less as best pleaseth the taste, sweeten it with Sugar, and drink a Wine draught in the morning, and at four a clock in the afternoon, and then walk and use some exercise after it. The party that hath the Scurvy, and whose legs are much swelled, may put into the drink some Juniper berries bruised, half an ounce, or thereabouts.

Dr. Bates *his Medicine against a Consumption.*

Take Liverwort two handfuls, Succory six, Endiffe, Borage, Colts-foot, of each six handfus, shred these finely, put them in a galon of new Milk, let them steep all night, in the morning
di-

distil them in a glass still, then take three spoonfuls of red Rose-water, three spoonfuls of this water; with half a pint of red Cows Milk, and as much Sugar of Rose as will sweeten it.

To make Gascony Powder.

Take the black tips of Crabs claws, gotten when the Sun is in *Cancer*, pick out from within them all the Fish, beat them to as fine a powder as you can, then searse it through a very fine searse, take an ounce of this powder, and put to it half an ounce of the Magestical of Pearl, and as much of the Magestical of Coral, mix them well together, then put a little Rose-water in a glass, in which you must hang a little Saffron in a bag, and a little Musk and Ambergrease in another; let them hang in Rose-water two or three dayes, till the vertue of them be gone into the water, then put your powder either into a Silver Porringer, or a white earthen one, and put as much of the Rose-water as will moisten your powder, then dry it in the Porringer by a gentle fire, and so wet your powder three or four times, and

as

as often dry it, after this make a Gely as followeth.

Take a Viper alive in *May* or *June*, cut off his head and tail, above the Navil pull off his skin, and with a clean cloth rub it dry, and so you may hang them up, and take two of those skins, and slice them small with a little Hartshorn; and make a Gelly of them, you need not make much, then when your powder is dry, wet it three or four times with this Gely, and as often dry it, and at last put no more Gelly then will moisten the powder; then make it up in balls as big and as little as you please, and dry them in a stove; and so keep them all the year.

Take of this Powder twelve or fourteen grains, either dry, or in a spoonful of small beer, in which there is a little Syrup of Clove-gilly-flowers.

Certain Plaisters, and their Uses.

1. *Emplast. Deminum* two pound; it is good for all kinde of bruises, or boils, or old sores, &c.

2. *Emplast. Mellilot* two pound; it is good for all sorts of green Wounds or bruises.

bruises or swellings, or to breed flesh being wanting.

3. *Diapalma* two pound; it is a very fine drying Plaister, and a good defensive to defend wounds from Inflamation, &c.

4. *Oxicroceum* four ounces; it is an extraordinary good warming Plaister for broken bones, or any cold cause, &c.

Certain Oyntments, and their Use.

1. *Unguentum Dialthea* one half pound; it is good to asswage pain, dissolve swellings or hardness.

2. *Unguentum Populeon*; it is a great cooling Oyntment for fire, or any great inflammation or any burning.

3. *Unguentum Album* six ounces; a fine cooling skining Oyntment to mix with others, &c.

4. *Unguentum Nervinum* four ounces; it is good for all cold causes of the Sinnews or Joynts.

5. *Unguentum Tutiæ* two ounces, good for watring sore Eyes.

6. *Unguentum Basilicon* seven ounces, good

good to fill hollow Ulcers with flesh, and apply a Plaister on the top of it.

7. Balsam two ounces good for all sorts of green wounds, being put in warm.

A Receipt of the Oyl of Johns-wort.

Take a quart of the best white Wine, infuse therein pickt flowers of Saint Johns-wort, then stow those flowers very dry, and put in more into the same Wine, infuse them again, so long that the Wine be very strong and red coloured with the Saint Johns-wort, then strain out the Wine clear from the flowers, put thereto a pint of the best Sallet Oyl, a quarter of an ounce of Cinnamon bruised, a quarter of Cloves bruised, one race of very good Ginger sliced, one good handful of the yellow flowers of Saint Johns-wort pickt very clean; boil all these on a very soft fire, till the Wine be all evaporated, when it is almost boiled, put in one good spoonful of pure Oyl of Turpentine, let that boil in it a little; so keep it for your use, the elder the better.

A Receipt for an extraordinary wasting of the Back, and for the Stone and Shrangury used by Justice Hutton.

Take Plantain and Ribwort, distill them in an ordinary Rose still, when you have occasion to use it, take Pippins and roast them, and take away the skin and core, and put them into the water, making thereof a lambswool as thick as you please, sweeten it with some Loaf sugar, the sweeter the better, take thereof half a pint when you go to bed, and this do nine or ten nights together, especially when you feel an heat in the Back.

For the Teeth.

If you will keep your teeth from rotting, or aching, wash the mouth continually every morning with juyce of Lemons, and afterward rub your teeth with a Sage leaf, and wash your teeth after meat with fair water.

To cure the Tooth-ache.

1. Take Mastick and chew it in your mouth till it is soft as Wax, then stop your teeth with it, if hollow there remaining till it is consumed, and it will certainly cure you.

2. The tooth of a dead man carried about a man, presently suppresses the pains of the teeth.

FINIS.

A QUEENS DELIGHGT:

OR,

The ART

OF

Preserving, *Conserving*, and *Candying*;

As also,

A right Knowledge of making PERFUMES, and Distilling the most Excellent Waters.

Never before Published.

Printed by *R. Wood* for *Nath. Brooks*, at the Angel in *Cornhill*, 1658.

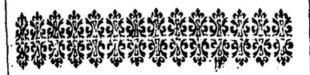

A Queens Delight:

OF

Conserves, and Preserves, Candying, and Distilling waters.

To preserve white Pear-plums or green.

Take the Plums, and cut the stalk off, and wipe them, then take the just weight of them in Sugar, then put them in a skillet of water, and let them stand in and scald, being close covered till they be tender, they must not seethe, when they be soft, lay them in a dish, and cover them with a cloth, and stew some of the sugar in the glass bottom, and p[ut] in the Plums, strewing the Sugar ove[r] till all be in, then let them stand all nigh[t] the next day put them in a pan; and le[t] them boil apace, keeping them clea[n] scummed, and when your Plums loo[k] clear, your syrup will gelly, and the[y] are enough. If your Plums be ripe, pee[l] off the skins before you put them in th[e] glass; they will be the better and clear[-] er a great deal to dry, if you will tak[e] the Plums white; if green, do them wit[h] the rines on.

To preserve Grapes.

Take Grapes when they be almo[st] through ripe, and cut the stalks off, an[d] stone them in the side, and as fast as yo[u] can stone them, strew sugar on them; yo[u] must take to every pound of Gra[pes] three quarters of a pound of Suga[r] then take some of the sower Grape[s] and wring the juyce of them, and put t[o] every pound of Grapes two spoonfu[ls] of juyce, then set them on the fire, a[nd] still lift up the pan and shake it roun[d] for fear of burning to, then set the[m] on again, and when the Sugar is mel[ted] ed, boil them as fast as you can possibly, and when they look very clear, and the syrup somewhat thick, they are enough.

To preserve Quinces white.

Take a pair and coar them, and to every pound of your equal weights in Sugar and Quince, take a wine pint of water; put them together, and boil them as fast as you can uncovered; and this way you may also preserve Pippins white as you do Quinces.

To preserve Respass.

Take a pound of Respass, a pound of fine Sugar, a quarter of a pint of the juyce of Respass, strew the sugar under and above the Respass, sprinkle the juyce all on them, set them on a clear fire, let them boil as soft as is possible, till the syrup will gelly, then take them of, let them stand till they be cold, then put them in a glass. After this manner is the best way.

To preserve Pippins.

Take fair Pippins, and boil them i[n]
fair water till they be somewhat tende[r]
then take them out, and peel off the skin
and put them into a fair earthen pot, an[d]
cover them till they be cold, then ma[ke]
the Syrup with fair water and Suga[r]
seethe it, and scum it very clean, then b[e]-
ing almost cold, put in your Pippins, [and]
boil them softly together, put in [as]
much rine of Oranges as you thi[nk]
will taste them, if you have no Oran[ges]
take whole Cinnamon and Cloves,
boil them high enough to keep them [all]
the year.

To preserve Fruits green.

Take Pippins, Apricocks, Pe[ars]
plums, or Peaches when they be gre[en]
scald them in hot water, and peel th[em]
or scrape them, put them into anoth[er]
water not so hot as the first, then b[oil]
them very tender, take the weight [of]
them in Sugar, put to it as much wa[ter]
as will make a Syrup to cover the[m]
then boil them something leasure[ly]

and take them up, then boil the Syrup till it be somewhat thick, that it will batten on a dish side, and when they are cold, put them together.

To preserve Oranges and Lemmons the best Way.

Take and boil them as for paste, then take as much Sugar as they weigh, and put to it as much water as will cover them by making a Syrup, then boil them very leasurely till they be clear, then take them up, and boil the Syrup till it batten on the dish side, and when they are cold put them up, &c.

An approved Conserve for a Cough or Consumption of the Lungs.

Take a pound of Elecampane roots, draw out the pith, and boil them in two waters, till they be soft, when it is cold put to it the like quantity of the pap of roasted Pippins, and three times their weight of brown Sugar-candy beaten to powder; stamp these in a Mortar to a Conserve, whereof take every morning fasting as much as a Walnut for a week or fortnight together, and afterwards but three times a week. *Approved.*

To make a Conserve of any of these Fruits.

When you have boiled your paste as followeth, ready to fashion on the Pie-plate, put it up into Gallipots, and never dry it, and this is all the difference between Conserves. And so you may make Conserves of any Fruits, this for all hard fruits, as Quinces, Pippins, Oranges and Lemons.

To dry any Fruits after they are preserved or Candy them.

Take Pippins, Pears, or Plums, and wash them out in warm water from the syrup they are preserved in, strew them over with searsed sugar, as you would do flower upon fish to fry them; set them in a broad earthen pan, that they may lie one by one; then set them in a warm oven or Stove to dry. If you will candy them withal, you must strew on sugar three or four times in the drying.

To preserve Artichokes young, green Walnuts and Lemons, and the Elecampane roots, or any bitter thing.

Take any of these, and boil them tender, and shift them in their boiling six or seven times to take away their bitterness, out of one hot water into another, then put a quart of Salt unto them, then take them up and dry them with a fair cloth, then put them into as much clarified Sugar as will cover them then let them boil a walm or two, and so let them stand soaking in the Sugar till the next morning, then take them up, and boil the Sugar a little higher by it self, and when they are cold put them up.

Let your green Walnuts be prickt full of holes with a great pin, and let them not be long in one water, for that will make them look black; being boiled tender, stick two or three Cloves in each of them.

Set your Elecampane roots, being clean scraped, and shifted in their boilings a dozen times, then dry them in a fair cloth, and so boil them as is
above

above written, take half so much more then it doth weigh, because it is bitter, &c.

To preserve Quinces white or red.

Take the Quinces, and coar them, and pare them, those that you will have white, put them into a pale of water two or three hours, then take as much Sugar as they weigh, put to it as much water as will make a Syrup to cover them, then boil your Syrup a little while, then put your Quinces in, and boil them as fast as you can, till they be tender and clear, then take them up, and boil the Syrup a little higher by it self, and being cold put them up. And if you will have them red, put them raw into Sugar, and boil them leasurely close covered till they be red, and put them not into cold water.

To preserve Grapes.

Take the Clusters, and stone them as you do Barberries, then take a little more Sugar then they weigh, put to it as much Apple water as will make a
Syrup

Syrup to cover them, then boil them as you do Cherries, as fast as you can, till the Syrup be thick, and being cold, pot it. Thus may you preserve Barberries or English Currans, or any kinde of Berries.

To preserve Pippins, Apricocks, Pearplums, and Peaches when they are ripe.

Take Pippins and pare them, bore a hole through them, and put them into a pale of water, then take as much Sugar as they do weigh, and put it to as much water as will make a Syrup to cover them, and boil them as fast as you can, so that you keep them from breaking, until they be tender, that you may prick a rush through them; let them be a soaking till they be almost cold, then put them up.

Your Apricocks and Peaches must be stoned, and not pared, but the Pearplums must not be stoned nor pared. Then take a little more Sugar then they weigh, then take as much Apple-water and Sugar as will make a Syrup for them, then boil them as you do your Pippins, and pot them as you do the Pippins likewise, &c.

To preserve Pippins, Apricocks, Pear-plums, or Peaches green.

Take you Pippins green and quoddle them in fair water, but let the water boil first before you put them in, and you must shift them in two hot waters before they will be tender, then pull off the skin from them, and so case them in so much clarified sugar as will cover them, and so boil them as fast as you can, keeping them from breaking, then take them up, and boil the syrup until it be as thick as for Quiddony; then pot them, and pour the sirup into them before they be cold.

Take your Apricocks and Pear-plums, and boil them tender, then take as much sugar as they do weigh, and take as much water as will make the syrup, take your green Peaches before they be stoned, and thrust a pin through them, and then make a strong water of ashes, and cast them into the hot standing lie to take off the fur from them, then wash them in three or four waters warm, so then put them into so much clarified sugar as will candy them; so boil them, and put them up, &c.

To dry Pippins or Pears without Sugar.

Take Pippins or Pears and prick them full of holes with a bodkin, and lay them in sweet wort three or four dayes, then lay them on a sieves bottom till they be dry in an Oven, but a drying heat. This you may do to any tender Plum.

To make Syrup of Clove-gilly-flowers.

Take a quart of water, half a bushel of Flowers, cut off the whites, and with a Sieve sift away the seeds, bruise them a little; let your water be boiled, and a little cold again, then put in your Flowers, and let them stand close covered twenty four hours; you may put in but half the flowers at a time, the strength will come out the better; to that liquor put in three pound of Sugar, let it lie in all night, next day boil it in a Gallipot, set it in a pot of water, and there let it boil till all the Sugar be melted, and the Syrup be pretty thick, then take it out, and let it stand in that till it be through cold, then glass it.

To make Syrup of Hysop for Colds.

Take a handful of Hysop, of Figs, Raisins, Dates, of each an ounce, of Collipint half an handful, French Barley one ounce, boil therein three pints of fair water to a quart, strain it and clarifie it with two whites of Eggs, then put in two pound of fine Sugar, and boil it to a syrup.

To make Orange Water.

Take a pottle of the best Malligo Sack, and put in as many of the peels of Oranges as will go in, cut the white clean off, let them steep twenty four hours; still them in a Glass still, and let the water run into the receiver upon fine Sugarcandy; you may still it in an ordinary still.

To dry Cherries.

Take a pound of sugar, dissolve it in thin fair water, when it is boiled a little while, put in your Cherries after they are stoned, four pound to one pound of sugar; let them lie in the sugar three dayes, then take them out of the syrup and lay them on sives one by one, and set them before the sun upon stools, turn them every day, else they will mould when they look of a dark red colour, and are dry, then put them up. And so you may do any manner of fruit In the sun is the best drying of them; put into the syrup some juyce of Rasps.

To make Juyce of Liquorish

Take English Liquorish, and stamp it very clean, bruise it with a hammer, and cut it in small pieces; to a pound of Liquorish thus bruised, put a quart of Hysop-water, let them soak together in an earthen pot a day and a night, then pull the Liquorish into small pieces, and lay it in soak again two dayes more; then strain out the Liquorish, and boil the liquor a good while. Stir it often, then put in half a pound of Sugar-candy, or Loaf Sugar finely beaten, four grains of Musk, as much Ambergreese, bruise them small with a little Sugar; then boil them together till it be good and thick, still have a care you

you burn it not; then put it out in glass plates, and make it into round rolls, and set it in a drying place till it be stiff, that you may work it into rolls to be cut as big as Barley corns, and so lay them on a place again: If it be needful strew on the place a little Sugar to prevent thickning; so dry them still if there be need, and if they should be too dry, the heat of the fire will soften them again.

A Perfume for Clothes, Gloves.

Take of Linet two grains, of Musk three, of Ambergreese four, and the Oyl of Bems a pretty quantity; grinde them all upon a Marble stone fit for that purpose; then with a brush or spunge, rake them over, and it will sweeten them very well; your Gloves or Jerkins must first be washed in old red Rose-water, and when they are almost dry, stretch them forth smooth, and lay on the Perfumes.

To make Almond Bisket.

Take the whites of four new laid Eggs,

Eggs, and two yolks, then beat it well for an hour together, then have in readiness a quarter of a pound of the best Almonds blanched in cold water, and beat them very small with Rosewart for fear of Oyling; then have a pound of the best Loaf Sugar finely beaten, beat that in the Eggs a while, then put in your Almonds, and five or six spoonfuls of the finest flower, and so bake them together upon paper or plates, you may have a little fine sugar in a piece of Tiffany to dust them over as they be in the Oven, so bake them as you do Bisket.

To make Conserve of Roses boiled.

Take a quart of red Rose-water, a quart of fair water, boil in the water a pound of red Rose leaves, the whites cut off, the leaves must be boiled very tender; then take three pound of Sugar, and put to it a pound at a time, and let it boil a little between every pound, so put it up in your pots.

To make Conserves of Roses, unboiled.

Take a pound of red Rose leaves, the whites cut off, stamp them very fine, take a pound of Sugar, and beat in with the Roses, and put it in a pot, and cover it with leather, and set it in a cool place.

To dry Apricocks.

First stone them, then weigh them, take the weight of them in double refined Sugar, make the syrup with so much water as will wet them, and boil it up so high, that a drop being dropped on a Plate it will slip clean off, when it is cold; then put in your Apricocks being pared, whilst your syrup is hot, but it must not be taken off the fire before you put them in, then turn them in the syrup often, then let them stand three quarters of an hour; then take them out of the syrup, and tie them up in Tiffanies, one in a Tiffany or more, as they be in bigness, and whilst you are tying them up, set the syrup on the fire to heat, but not to boil, then put
your

your Apricocks into the syrup, and set them on a quick fire, and let them boil as fast as you can, skim them clean, and when they look clear, take them from the fire, and let them lie in the syrup till the next day, then set them on the fire to heat, but not to boil; then set them by till the next day, and lay them upon a clean Sieve to drain, and when they are well drained, take them out of the Tiffanies, and so dry them in a stove, or better in the sun with glasses over them, to keep them from the dust.

To make Quinces for Pies.

Wipe the Quinces, and put them into a little vessel of small beer when it hath done working; stop them close that no air can get in, and this will keep them fair all the year, and good.

The best way to break sweet Powder.

Take of Orrice one pound, Calamus a quarter of a pound, Benjamin one half pound, Storax half a pound, Civet a quarter of an ounce, Cloves a quarter of of a pound, Musk one half ounce, Oyl of Orange flowers one ounce, Lignum Aloes one ounce, Rosewood a quarter of a pound, Ambergreese a quarter of an ounce. To every pound of Roses put a pound of Powder; the bag must be of Taffaty, or else the powder will run through.

To make excellent Perfumes.

Take a quarter of a pound of Damask Rose-buds cut clean from the Whites, stamp them very small, put to them a good spoonful of Damask Rose-water, so let them stand close stopped all night, then take one ounce and a quarter of Benjamin finely beaten, and also searsed, (if you will) twenty grains of Civit, and ten grains of Musk; mingle these with the Roses, beating them well together, then make it up in little Cakes between Rose leaves, and dry them between sheets of paper.

To make a very good Pomatum.

Take the fat of a young Dog one pound, it must be killed well, that the blood

blood settle not into the fat, then let the outer skin be taken off before it be opened, lest any of the hair come to the fat, then take all the fat from the inside, and assoon as you take it off fling it into Conduit-water; and if you see the second skin be clear, peel it, and water it with the other; be sure it cools not out of the water: you must not let any of the flesh remain on it, for then the Pomatum will not keep. To one pound of this fat take two pound of Lambs caule, and put it to the other in the water, and when you see it is cold, drain it from the water in a Napkin, and break it in little pieces with your fingers, and take out all the little veins; then take eight ounces of Oyl of Tartar, and put in that first, stirring it well together, then put it into a Gallon of Conduit-water, and let it stand till night; shift this with so much Oyl and Water, morning and evening seven dayes together, and be sure you shift it constantly; and the day before you mean to melt it, wring it hard by a little at a time, and be sure the Oyl and Water be all out of it, wring the water well out of it with a Napkin every time you shift it; then put

put in three pints of Rose-water; let it stand close covered twelve hours; then wring out that, and put in a pint of fresh Rose-water into a high Gallipot with the feces; then tie it close up, and set it in a pot of water, and let it boil two hours, then take it out, and strain it into an earthen pan, let it stand till it is cold; then cut a hole in it, and let out the water, then scrape away the bottom, and dry it with a cloth, and dry the pan; melt it in a Chafing-dish of coals, or in the Gallipots; beat it so long, till it look very white and shining; then with your hand fling it in fine Cakes upon white paper, and let it lie till it be cold, then put it into Gallipots. This will be very good for two or three years.

To make Raisin Wine.

Take two pound of Raysins of the Sun shred, a pound of good powdered Sugar, the juyce of two Lemons, one pill; put these in an earthen pot with a top, then take two galons of water, let it boil half an hour, then take it hot from the fire, and put it into the pot, and
cover

cover it close for three or four dayes, stirring it twice a day, being strained put it into bottles, and stop it very close; In a fortnight or three weeks it may be drunk; you may put in Cloves, Gillyflowers, or Cowslips, as the time of the year is when you make it; and when you have drawn this from the Raysins, and bottled it up, heat two quarts of water more, put it to the Ingredients, and let it stand as aforesaid. This will be good, but smaller then the other, the water must be boiled as the other.

To make Rasberry Wine.

Take a Gallon of good Rhennish Wine, put into it as much Rasberries very ripe as will make it strong, put it in an earthen pot, and let it stand two days; then pour your Wine from your Rasberries, and put into every bottle two ounces of Sugar. Stop it up, and keep it by you.

The best way to preserve Cherries.

Take the best Cherries you can get, and cut the stalks something short, then
for

for every pound of these Cherries take two pound of other Cherries, and put them off their stalks and stones, put to them ten spoonfuls of fair water, and then set them on the fire to boil very fast till you see that the colour of the Syrup be like pale Claret Wine, then take it off the fire, and drain them from the Cherries into a pan to preserve in. Take to every pound of Cherries a quarter of sugar, of which take half, and dissolve it with the Cherry-water drained from the Cherries, and keep them boiling very fast till they will gelly in a spoon, and as you see the syrup thin, take off the sugar that you kept finely beaten, and put it to the Cherries in the boiling; the faster they boil, the better they will be preserved, and let them stand in a pan till they be almost cold.

A Tincture of Ambergreese.

Take Ambergreese one ounce, Musk two drams, spirit of Wine half a pint, or as much as will cover the Ingredients two or three fingers breadth, put all into a glass, stop it close with a cork and bladder, set it in Horse dung ten or twelve

twelve dayes, then pour off gently the spirit of Wine, and keep it in a glass close stopt; then put more spirit of Wine on the Ambergreese, and do as before, then pour it off, after all this the Ambergreese will serve for ordinary uses. A drop of this will perfume any thing, and in Cordials it is very good.

To make Usquebath the best Way.

Take two quarts of the best *Aqua vitæ*, four ounces of scraped liquorish, and half a pound of sliced Raisins of the Sun, Anniseeds four ounces, Dates and Figs of each half a pound, sliced Nutmeg, Cinnamon, Ginger, of each half an ounce, put these to the *Aqua vitæ*, stop it very close, and set it in a cold place ten dayes, stirring it twice a day with a stick, then strain or sweeten it with Sugarcandy; after it is strained, let it stand till it be clear, then put into the glass Musk and Ambergreese; two grains is sufficient for this quantity.

To preserve Cherries with a quarter of their weight in Sugar.

Take four pound of Cherries, one pound

pound of Sugar, beat your Sugar and strew a little in the bottom of your skillet, then pull off the stalks and stones of your Cherries, and cut them cross the bottom with a knife; let the juyce of the Cherries run upon the Sugar; for there must be no other liquor but the juyce of the Cherries; cover your Cherries over with one half of your Sugar. Boil them very quick; when they are half boiled, put in the remainder of your Sugar; when they are almost enough, put in the rest of the Sugar; you must let them boyl till they part in sunder like Marmalade, stirring them continually, so put them up hot into your warm Marmalade glasses.

To make Gelly of Pippins.

Take Pippins, and pare them, and q[uar]ter them, and put as much water to t[hem] as will cover them, and let them boi[l] till all the vertue of the Pippins are out then strain them, and take to a pint that liquor a pound of Sugar, and long threads of Orange peels, and in it, then take a Lemmon, and pare a slice it very thin, and boil it in your quor a little thin; take them out, and lay them in the bottom of your glass, and when it is boiled to a gelly, pour it on the Lemons in the glass. You must boil the Oranges in two or three waters before you boil it in the gelly.

To make Apricock Cakes.

Take the fairest Apricocks you can get, and parboil them very tender, then take off the pulp and their weight of Sugar, and boil the Sugar and Apricocks together very fast; stir them ever lest they burn to, and when you can see the bottom of the Skillet it is enough, then put them into Cards sowed round, and dust them with fine Sugar, and when they are cold stone them, then turn them, and fill them up with some more of the same stuff; but you must let them stand for three or four dayes before you turn them off the first place; and when you finde they begin to candy, take them out of the Cards, dust them with Sugar again; so do even when you turn them.

To preserve Barberries the best way.

First stone them and weigh them, half a pound of Sugar to half a pound of them, then pare them and slice them into that liquor, take the weight of it in Sugar; then take as many Rasberries as will colour it, and strain them into the liquor, then put in the sugar, boil it as fast as you can, then skim it till it be very clear, then put in your Barberries, and that sugar you weighed, and so let them boil till the skin be fully risen up, then take them off, and skin them very clean, and put them up.

To make Lozinges of red Roses.

Boil your sugar to sugar again, then put in your Red Roses being finely beaten, and made moist with the juyce of a Lemmon, let it not boil after the Roses are in, but pour it upon a Pye-plate, and cut it into what form you please.

To make Chips of Quinces.

First scald them very well, then slice them into a dish, and pour a Candy syrup to them scalding hot, and let them stand all night, then lay them on plates, and searse sugar on them, and turn them every day, and scrape more sugar on them till they be dry. If you would have them look clear, heat them in syrup, but not to boil.

To make Sugar of Wormwood, Mint, Anniseed, or any other of that kinde.

Take double refined Sugar, and do but wet it in fair water, or Rose-water, and boil it to a Candy, when it is almost boiled take it off, and stir it till it be cold, then drop in three or four drops of the Oyls of whatsoever you will make, and stir it well; then drop it on a board, being before sifted with Sugar.

To make Syrup of Lemons or Citrens.

Pare off all the rindes, then slice your Lemmons very thin, and lay a lare of sugar

Sugar finely beaten, and a Jare of Lemons in a silver Bason till you have fitted it, or as much as you mean to make, and so let it stand all night; the next day pour off the liquor that runs from it into a glass through a Tiffany strainer. Be sure you put Sugar enough to them at the first, and it will keep a year good, if it be set up well.

To make Jumbals of Apricocks or Quinces

Take Apricocks or Quinces, and quoddle them tender, then take their Pulp and dry it in a dish over a Chafing-dish of coals, and set it in a stove for a day or two; then beat it in a stone Mortar, putting in as much Sugar as will make a stiff paste; then colour it with Saunders, Cochinele or blew Starch, and make it up in what colour you please rowl them with battle-doors into long pieces, and tye them up in knots, and dry them

To make Cherry-water.

Take nine pound of Cherries, pull out the stones and stalks, break the with your hand, and put them into nine pints of Claret Wine, take nine ounces of Cinnamon, and three Nutmegs, bruise them, and put them into this, then take of Rosemary and Balm, of each half a handful, of sweet Marjoram a quarter of an handful; put all these with the aforenamed into an earthen pot well leaded, so let them stand to infuse twenty four hours, stirring it once in four or five hours; so distill it in a Limbeck, keeping the strongest water by it self, put some Sugar finely beaten into your glasses. If your first water be too strong, put some of the second to it as you use it. If you please you may tie some Musk, and Ambergreese in a rag, and hang it by a thread in your glass.

To make Orange Cakes.

Take Oranges and pare them as thin as you can, then take out the meats clean, and put them in water; let them lie about an hour, shift the water, and boil them very tender in three or four waters, then put them up, and dry them on a cloth: mince them as small as you can, then put them into a dish, and squeeze all the juyce of the meat into them, and

let them stand till the next day, take t
every pound of these a pound, and a
quarter of double refined Sugar; Boil
it with a spoonful of water at the bottom to keep it from burning till it be
Sugar again; then put in your Oranges,
and let them stand and dry on the fire
but not boil; then put them on glass
plates, and put them in a stove, the next
day make them into Cakes, and so dry
them as fast as you can.

To preserve Oranges the French way.

Take twelve of the fairest Oranges and
best coloured, and if you can get them
with smooth skins they are the better,
and lay them in Conduit water six days
and nights, shifting them into fresh water
morning and evening; then boil them very tender, and with a knife pare them very
thin, rub them with salt, when you have
so done, core them with a coring Iron
taking out the meat and seeds; then rub
them with a dry cloth till they be clean
and to every pound of Oranges a pound
and half of Sugar, and to a pound of Sugar a pint of water; then mingle your
sugar and water well together in a large
skillet or pan; beat the whites of three
Eggs

A Queens Delight.

Eggs, and put that into it, then set it on the fire, and let it boil till it rises, and strain it through a Napkin; then set it on the fire again, and let it boil till the syrup be thick, then put in your Oranges, and make them seethe as fast as you can, now and then putting in a piece of fine loaf sugar the bigness of a Walnut, when they have boiled near an hour, put into them a pint of Apple water: then boil them apace, and half a pint of white Wine, this should be put in before the Apple water, when your Oranges are very clear, and your syrup so thick that it will gelly, (which you may know by setting them to cool in a spoon) when they are ready to be taken off from the fire; then put in the juyce of eight Lemons warm into them, then put them into an earthen pan, and so let them stand till they be cold, then put every Orange in a several glass or pot, if you do but six Oranges at a time, it is the better.

To preserve Green Plums.

The greatest Wheaten Plum is the best, which will be ripe in the midst of July,

July, gather them about that time, or later, as they grow in bigness, but you must not suffer them to turn yellow, for then they never be of good colour; being gathered, lay them in water for the space of 12. hours, and when you gather them, wipe them with a clean linnen cloth, and cut off a little of the stalks of every one; then set two skillets of water on the fire, and when one is scalding hot put in your Plums, and take them from the fire, and cover them, and let them rest for the space of a quarter of an hour; then take them up; and when your other skillet of water doth boil, put them into it; let them but stay in it a very little while, and so let the other skillet of water, wherein they were first boiled, be set to the fire again, and make it to boil, and put in your plums as before, and then you shall see them rivet over, and yet your Plums very whole; then while they be hot, you must with your knife scrape away the rivetting; then take to every pound of Plums a pound and two ounces of Sugar finely beaten, then set a pan with a little fair water on the fire, and when it boils, put in your Plums, and let them seethe half a quarter of an hour till you see the colour wax green, then set them off the fire a quarter of an hour, and take a handful of Sugar that is weighed, and strow it in the bottom of the pan wherein you will preserve, and so put in your Plums one by one, drawing the liquor from them, and cast the rest of your sugar on them; then set the pan on a moderate fire, letting them boil continually but very softly, and in three quarters of an hour they will be ready, as you may perceive by the greenness of your Plums, and thickness of your Syrup, which if they be boiled enough, will gelly when it is cold; then take up your Plums, and put them into a Gallipot, but boil your Syrup a little longer, then strain it into some vessel, and being blood-warm, pour it upon your Plums, but stop not the pot before they be cold. Note also you must preserve them in such a pan, as they may lie one by another, and turn of themselves; and when they have been five or six dayes in the Syrup, that the Syrup grow thin, you may boil it again with a little Sugar, but put it not to your Plums till they be cold. They must have three scaldings, and one boiling.

To dry Plums.

Take three quarters of a pound of sugar to a pound of black Pear-plums, or Damsins, slit the Plums in the crest, lay a lay of Sugar with a lay of Plums, and let them stand all night, if you stone the Plums, fill up the place with Sugar, then boil them but gently till they be very tender, without breaking the skins; take them into an earthen or silver dish, and boil your syrup afterwards for a gelly, then pour it in your Plums scalding hot, and let them stand two or three dayes, then let them be put to the Oven after you draw your bread, so often until your syrup be dried up, and when you think they are almost dry, lay them in a sieve, and pour some scalding water on them, which will run through the Sieve, and set them in an Oven afterwards to dry.

To preserve Cherries the best way, bigger then they grow naturally, &c.

Take a pound of the smallest Cherries, and boil them tender in a pint o fair water, then strain the liquor from the substance, then take two pound of good Cherries, and put them in a preserving pan with a lay of Cherries, and a lay of Sugar, then pour the syrup of the other Cherries about them, and so let them boil as fast as you can with a quick fire, that the syrup may boil over them, and when your syrup is thick and of good colour, then take them up, and let them stand a cooling by partitions one from another, and being cold you may pot them up.

To preserve Damsins, red Plums or black.

Take your Plums newly gathered, and take a little more Sugar then they do weigh, then put to it as much water as will cover them; then boil your syrup a little while, and so let it cool, then put in your Damsins or plums, then boil them leasurely in a pot of seething water till they be tender, then being almost cold pot them up.

To dry Pippins or Pears.

Take your Pippins, Pears, Apricocks, pare

pare them, and lay them in a broad earthen pan one by one, and so rowl them in searsed Sugar as you flower fried fish; put them in an Oven as hot as for Manchet, and so take them out, and turn them as long as the Oven is hot; when the Oven is of a drying heat, lay them upon a paper, and dry them on the bottom of a Sieve; so you may do the least Plum that is.

To dry Pippins or Pears another way.

Take Pippins or Pears, and lay them in an earthen pan one by one, and when they be baked plump and not broken, then take them out, and lay them up, and lay them upon a paper, then lay them on a Sieves bottom, and dry them as you did before.

To dry Apricocks tender.

Take the ripest of the Apricocks, pare them, put them into a silver or earthen skillet, and to a pound of Apricocks put three quarters of a pound of Sugar, set your Apricocks over your fire, stiring them till they come to a pulp, and
set

set the Sugar in another skillet by boiling it up to a good height, then take all the Apricocks, and stir them round till they be well mingled, then let it stand till it be something cold and thick, then put it into Cards, being cut of the fashion of an Apricock, and laid upon glass plates; fill the Cards half full, then set them in your Stove; but when you finde they are so dry that they are ready to turn, then provide as much of your pulp as you had before, and to put to every one a stove when they are turned, (which you must have said before) and pour the rest of the Pulp upon them, so set them into your stove, turning them till they be dry.

To dry Plums.

Take a pound of Sugar to a pound of Plums, pare them, scald your Plums, then lay your Plums upon a sieve till the water be drained from them, boil your Sugar to a Candy height, and then put your Plums in whilest your Syrup is hot, so warm them every morning for a week, then take them out, and put them into your stove and dry them.

To dry Apricocks.

Take your Apricocks, pare and stone them, then weigh half a pound of Sugar to a pound of Apricocks, then take half that sugar, and make a thin Syrup, and when it boileth, put in the Apricocks, then scald them in that Syrup; then take them off the fire, and let them stand all night in that syrrup, in the morning take them out of that Syrup, and make another Syrup with the other half of the Sugar, then put them in, and preserve them till they look clear; but be sure you do not do them so much as those you keep preserved without drying; then take them out of that Syrup, and lay them on a piece of plate till they be cold; then take a skillet of fair water, and when the water boils take your Apricocks one after another in a spoon, and dip them in the water first on one side, and then on the other; not letting them go out of the spoon: you must do it very quick; then put them on a piece of a plate, and dry them in a stove, turning them every day, you must be sure that your Stove or Cubboard

board where you dry them, the heat of it be renewed three times a day with a temperate drying heat until they be something dry, then afterwards turn once as you see cause.

Conserves of Violets the Italian manner.

Take the leaves of blew Violets separated from their stalks and greens, beat them very well in a stone Mortar, with twice their weight of Sugar, and reserve them for your use in a glass vessel.

The Vertue.

The heat of Choler it doth mitigate, extinguisheth thirst, asswageth the Belly, and helpeth the Throat of hot hurts, sharp droppings and dryness, and procureth rest, It will keep one year.

Conserves of red Roses the Italian manner.

Take fresh red Roses not quite ripe, beat them in a stone Mortar, mix them with double their weight of Sugar, and put them in a glass close stopped, being not full, let them remain before you use them three moneths, stirring of them once a day.

The

The Vertue.

The Stomach, Heart, and Bowels it cooleth, and hindereth vapours, the spitting of blood and corruption for the most part (being cold) it helpeth. It will keep many years.

Conserve of Borage Flowers after the Italian Manner.

Take fresh Borage flowers cleansed well from their heads four ounces, fine Sugar twelve ounces, beat them well together in a stone Mortar, and keep them in a vessel well placed.

The Vertues are the same with Bugloss flowers.

Conserve of Rosemary Flowers after the Italian Manner.

Take new Rosemary Flowers one pound, of white Sugar one pound; so beat them together in a Marble Mortar with a wooden Pestle, keep it in a Gallipot, or vessel of earth well glassed, or in one of hard stone. It may be preserved for one year or two.

A Queens Delight. 235

The Vertues.

It comforteth the Heart, the Stomach, the Brain, and all the nervous parts of the Body.

Conserve of Betony after the Italian Way.

Betony new and tender one pound, the best Sugar three pound, beat them very small in a stone Mortar, let the Sugar be boiled with two pound of Betony-water to the consistence of a syrup, at length mix them together by little and little over a small fire, and make a Conserve, which keep in a glass.

The Vertues.

It helpeth the cold pains of the Head, purgeth the Stomach and Womb, it helpeth stoniness of the Reins, and furthereth Conception.

Conserve of Sage.

Take new flowers of Sage one pound, Sugar one pound; so beat them together very small in a Marble Mortar, put them in a vessel well glassed and leeped, set them in the Sunn, stir them

them daily; it will last one year.
The Vertues.

It is good in all cold hurts of the brain, it refresheth the Stomach, it openeth obstructions, and takes away superfluous and hurtful humours from the Stomach.

Conserve of the Flowers of Lavender.

Take the flowers being new, so many as you please, and beat them with three times their weight of white sugar, after the same manner as Rosemary flowers, they will keep one year.

The Vertues.

The Brain, the Stomach, Liver Spleen and Womb it maketh warm, and is good in the suffocation of the Womb, hardness of the Spleen, and for the Apoplex.

Conserve of Marjoram.

The Conserve is prepared as Betony, it keepeth a year.

The Vertues.

It is good against the coldness moistness of the Brain, and Stomach an and it strengtheneth the Vital Spirits.

Conserve of Piony after the Italian way.

In the Spring take of the flowers fresh half a pound, sugar one pound, beat them together in a good stone Mortar, then put them in a glass, and set them in the sun for three moneths, stirring them daily with a wooden spathula.

The Vertues.
It is good against the Falling-sickness, and giddiness of the Head, it cleanseth the Reins and Bladder.

Touching Candies, as followeth.

To Candy Rosemary flowers in the Sun.

TAke Gum Dragon, and steep it in Rose-water, then take the Rosemary

mary flowers, good coloured, and well pickt, and wet them in the water that your Gum Dragon is steeped in, then take them out, and lay them upon a Paper, and strew fine Sugar over them; this do in the hot Sun, turning them, and strewing Sugar on them, till they are candied, and so keep them for your use.

To make Sugar of Roses.

Take the deepest coloured red Roses, pick them, cut off the white buttons, and dry your red leaves in an Oven, till they be as dry as possible, then beat them to powder and searse them, then take half a pound of Sugar beaten fine, put it into your Pan with as much fair water as will wet it; then set it in a chafing-dish of coals, and let it boil till it be Sugar again; then put as much Powder of Roses that will make it look very red, stir them well together, and when it is almost cold, put it into Pales, and when it is throughly cold, take them off, and put them in boxes.

To Candy Pippins, Pears, Apricocks, or Plums.

Take any of these fruits being pared, and strew upon them, as you do flower upon frying fish, then lay them on a board in a Pewter dish, so put them into an Oven as hot as for Manchet; as the liquor comes from them, pour forth, turn them, and strew more Sugar on them, and sprinkle Rose-water on them, thus turning and sugaring of them three or four times, till they be almost dry, then lay them on a Lettice Wire, or on the bottom of a sieve in a warm oven, after the bread is drawn out, till they be full dry: so you may keep them all the year.

To Candy or Clear Rockandy Flowers.

Take spices, and boil them in a syrup of sugar, then put in the flowers, boil them till they be stiff; when you spread them on a paper, lay them on round Wiers in an earthen pan, then take as much hard Sugar as will fill your pan, and as much water as will melt the Sugar,

gar, that is half a pint to every pound, then beat a dozen spoonfuls of fair water, and the white of an Egg in a bason, with a Birchin rod till it come to a froth, when your sugar is all melted and boiled, put the froth of the Egg in the hot syrup, and as it riseth, drop in a little cold water; so let it boil a little while, then scum it, then boil it to a Candy height, that is, when you may draw it in small threads between your finger and your thumb: then pour forth all your syrup that will run from it in your pan, then set it a drying one hour or two; which done, pick up the wiers, and take off the flowers, and lay them on papers, and so dry them.

To Candy Spanish flowers.

Take the Blossoms of divers sorts of flowers, and make a syrup of water and sugar, and boil it very thick, then put in your blossoms, and stir them in their boiling, till it turn to sugar again, then stir them with the back of a spoon, till the sugar fall from it; so may you keep them for sallets all the year.

To candy Grapes, Cherries or Barberries.

Take any of these fruits, and strew fine sifted sugar on them, as you do flower on frying fish, lay them on a lettice of wier in a deep earthen pan, and put them into an Oven as hot as for Manchet; then take them out, and turn them, and sugar them again, and sprinkle a little Rose-water on them. pour the syrup forth as it comes from them, thus turning and sugaring them till they be almost dry, then take them out of the earthen pan, and lay them on a lettice of wier upon two billets of Wood in a warm Oven, after the bread is drawn, till they by dry and well candied.

To candy Suckets of Oranges, Lemons, Citrons, and Angelica.

Take, and boil them in fair water tender, and shift them in three boilings, six or seven times, to take away their bitterness, then put them into as much sugar as will cover them, and so let them boil a walm or two, then take hem out, and dry them in a warm oven as hot as Manchet, and being dry, boil the Sugar to a Candy height, and so cast your Oranges into the hot Sugar, and take them out again suddenly, and then lay them upon a lettice of wier on the bottom of a sieve in a warm oven after the bread is drawn, still warming the Oven till it be dry, and they will be well candied.

To Candy the Orange roots.

Take the Orange roots being well and tenderly boiled, petch them and peel them, and wash them out of two or three waters; then dry them well with a fair cloth, then pot them together two or three in a knot, then put them into as much clarified Sugar as will cover, and so let them boil leasurely, turning them until you see the Sugar drunk up into the root, then shaking them in the Bason to sunder the knots; and when they wax dry, take them up suddenly, and lay them on sheets of white Paper, and so dry them before the fire an hour or two, and they will be well candied.

Candy Orange Peels after the Italian way.

Take Orange peels, so often steeped in cold water, as you think convenient for their bitterness, then dry them gently, and candy them with some convenient syrup made with Sugar; some that are more grown, take away that spongious white under the yellow peels, others do both together.

The Vertues.

They corroborate the Stomach and Heart.

To Candy Citrons after the Spanish way.

Take Citron Peels so large as you please, the inner part being taken away, let them be steeped in a clear lay of water and ashes for nine dayes, and shift them the fifth day, afterward wash them in fair water, till the bitterness be taken away, and that they grow sweet, then let them be boiled in fair water till they grow soft, the watery part being taken away, let them be steeped in a vessel of stone twenty four hours, with a Julip made of white Sugar, and three parts water,

water, after let them be boiled upon a gentle fire, to candness of Penidies or Paste; being taken out of that, let them be put in a glass vessel, one by one, with the Julip of Roses made somewhat hard, or with sugar; some do adde Amber and Musk to them.

The Virtues.

It comforteth the Stomach and Heart; it helpeth concoction.

Canded Cherries the Italian way.

Take Cherries before they are full ripe, the stones taken out, put clarified sugar boiled to a height, then pour it on them.

Chicory roots canded the Italian way.

Take Chicory new and green, the outward bark being taken away, then before they be canded, let them be cut in several parts, and gently boiled, that no bitterness may remain, then set them in the air placed severally, and put Sugar to them boiled to a height.

Touching Marmalets, and Quiddony, as followeth.

To make Marmalet of Damsins

TAke two quarts of Damsins that be through ripe, and pare off the skins of three pints of them, then put them into an earthen Pipkin, those with the skins undermost; then set the Pipkin into a pot of seething water, and let the water seethe apace until the Damsins be tender. Cover the Pipkin close, that no water get into them, and when they are tender, put them out into an earthen pan, and take out all the stones and skins, then weigh them, and take the weight with hard Sugar, then break the Sugar fine, and put it into the Damsins, then set it on the fire, and make it boil apace till it will come from the bottom of the skillet, then take it up, and put it into a glass, but scum it clear in the boiling.

To make white Marmalet of Quinces.

Take unpared Quinces, and boil them whole in fair water, peel them and take all the pap from the coar, to every pound thereof adde three quarters of a pound of Sugar, boil it well till it come well from the pans bottom, then put it into boxes.

To make Marmalet of any tender Plum.

Take your Plums, and boil them between two dishes on a Chafing-dish of coals, then strain it, and take as much Sugar as the Pulp do weigh, and put to it as much Rose water, and fair water as will melt it, that is, half a pint of water to a pound of Sugar, and so boil it to a Candy height, then put the pulp into hot Sugar, with the pap of a roasted apple. In like manner you must put roasted Apples to make Paste Royal of it, or else it will be tough in the drying.

To make Orange Marmalet.

Take Oranges, pare them as thin as you can, boil them in four several waters, let them be very soft before you take them out, then take two quarts of Spring-water, put thereto twenty Pippins pared, quartered and coared, let them boil till all the vertue be out; take heed they do not lose the colour; then strain them, put to every pint of water a pound of Sugar, boil it almost to a Candy height, then take out all the meat out of the Oranges, slice the peel in long slits as thin as you can, then put in your peel with the juyce of two Lemmons, and one half Orange, then boil it to a Candy.

To make Quiddeny of Pippins, of Ruby, or any Amber colour.

Take Pippins, and cut them in quarters, and pare them, and boil them with as much fair water as will cover them, till they be tender, and sunk into the water, then strain all the liquor from the Pulp, then take a pint of that liquor,

quor and half a pound of sugar, and boil it till it be a quaking gelly on the back of a spoon; so then pour it on your moulds, being taken out of fair water; then being cold, turn them on a wet trencher, and so slide them into the boxes, and if you would have it ruddy colour, then boil it leasurely close covered, till it be as red as Claret Wine, so may you conceive, the difference is in the boiling of it, remember to boil your Quinces in Apple-water as you do your Plums.

To make Quiddony of all kindes of Plums.

Take your Apple-water, and boil the Plums in it till it be red as Claret Wine, and when you have made it strong of the Plums, put to every pint half a pound of Sugar, and so boil it till a drop of it hang on the back of a spoon like a quaking gelly. If you will have it of an Amber colour, then boil it with a quick fire, that is all the difference of the colouring of it.

To make Marmalet of Oranges, or Orange Cakes, &c.

Take the yellowest and fairest Oranges, and water them three dayes, shifting the water twice a day, pare them as thin as you possible can, boil them in a water changed five or six times, until the bitterness of the Orange be boiled out; those that you preserve must be cut in halfs, but those for Marmalet must be boiled whole, let them be very tender, and slice them very thin on a trencher, taking out the seeds and long strings, and with a knife make it as fine as the Pap of an Apple; then weigh your Pap of Oranges, and to a pound of it, take a pound and half of Sugar: then you must have Pippins boiled ready in a skillet of fair water, and take the Pap of them made fine on a trencher, and the strings taken out, (but take not half so much Pippins as Oranges) then take the weight of it in sugar, and mix it both together in a silver or earthen dish; and set it on the coals to dry the water out of it, (as you do with Quince Marmalet) when your Sugar is Candy height; put in your stuff, and boil it till you think it stiff enough, stirring it continually, if you please you may put in a little Musk in it.

Touching Pastrey and Pasties.

To make Sugar cakes.

TAke three pound of the finest Wheat Flower, one pound of fine Sugar; Cloves, and Mace, of each one ounce finely searsed, two pound of Butter, a little Rose-water, knead and mould this very well together, melt your Butter as you put it in, then mould it with your hand forth upon a board, cut them round with a glass, then lay them on papers, and set them in an Oven, be sure you

Oven be not too hot, so let them stand till they be coloured enough.

To make clear cakes of Plums.

Take Plums of any sorts, Raspiss are the best, put them into a stone Jug, into a pot of seething water, and when they are dissolved, strain them together through a fair cloth, and take to a pint of that a pound of Sugar, put to as much colour as will melt it, and boil to a Candy height; boil the liquor likewise in another Posnet, then put them seething hot together, and so boil a little while stirring them together, then put them into glasses, and set them in an Oven or Stove in a drying heat, let them stand so two or three weeks, and never be cold, removing them from one warm place to another, they will turn in a week; beware you set them not too hot, for they will be tough; so every day turn them till they be dry; they will be very clear.

To make Paste of Oranges and Lemons.

Take your Oranges well coloured, boil

boil them tender in water, changing them six or seven times in the boiling, put into the first water one handful of Salt, and then beat them in a wooden Bowl with a wooden pestle, and then strain them through a piece of Cushion Canvas, then take somewhat more then the weight of them in sugar, then boil it, dry and fashion it as you please.

To make Rasberry Cakes.

Take Rasberries, and put them into a Gallipot, cover them close, and set them into a skillet of water, and let them boil till they are all to mash, then rub them through a strainer of Cushion Canvas, put the liquor into a silver bason, and set it upon a very quick fire, and put into it one handful or two of whole Rasberries, according to the quantity of your liquor: and as you shall like to have seeds in your Paste. Thus let it boil very fast till it be thick, and continually stir, lest it burn, then take two silver dishes that are of a weight, and put them into your scales, in the one put the Raspiss stuff, and in the other double refined Sugar finely beaten

beaten, as much as the weight of Raspiss stuff; then put as much water to the Sugar as will melt it, set it upon the fire, and let it boil till it be very high canded, then take it from the fire, and put your Raspiss stuff into it; and when your sugar and Rasberries are very well mixt together, and the Sugar all melted from about the dish (which if it will not do from the fire, set it on again) but let it not boil in any case; when it is pretty cool, lay it by spoonfuls in plates, and put it into your stuff, keeping temperate fire to it twice a day till it be canded that will; turn them, joyn two of the pieces together, to make the cake the thicker.

To make Paste of Genoa Citrons.

Take Citrons, and boil them in their skins, then scrape all the pulp from the coar, strain it through a piece of Cushion Canvas, take twice the weight of the Pulp in Sugar, put to it twice as much water as will melt it, that is half a pint to every pound of Sugar, boil it to a candy height; dry the Pulp upon a Chafing-Dish of Coals, then put the

the syrup and the Pulp hot together, boil it with stirring until it will lie upon a Pie-plate, set it in a warm stone Oven upon two billets of wood, from the heat of the Oven, all one night, in the morning turn it, and set it in the like heat again, so turn it every day till it be dry.

To make a French Tart.

Take a quartern of Almonds or thereabouts, and peel them, then beat them in a Mortar, take the white of the breast of a cold Capon, and take so much Lard as twice the quantity of the Capon, and so much Butter, or rather more, and half a Marrow bone, and if the bone be little then all the Marrow, with the juyce of one Lemon; beat them all together in a Mortar very well, then put in one half pound of loaf sugar grated, then take a good piece of Citron, cut it in small pieces, and half a quarter of Pistanius; mingle all these together, take some flower, and the yolks of two or three eggs, and some sweet Butter, and work it with cold water.

To make cakes of Pear-plums.

Take to a pound of the clear, or the Pulp, a pound of Sugar, and boil it to a Sugar again, then break it as small as you can, and put in the clear, when your sugar is well melted in it, and almost cold, put it in glass plates, and set them into your stove as fast as you can, with coals under them, and so twice a day whilest they be dry enough to cut; if you make them of the clear, you must make Paste of Apples to lay upon them, you must scald them, and beat them very well, and so use them as you do your Plums, and then you may put them into what fashion you please.

To make cakes: viz.

Take a pound of sugar finely beaten, four yolks of Eggs, two whites, one half pound of Butter washt in Rose-water, six spoonfuls of sweet Cream warmed, one pound of Currans well pickt, as much flower as will make it up, mingle them well together, make them into Cakes, bake them in an Oven, almost

most as hot as for manchet, half an hour will bake them.

To make a Cake the way of the Royal Princess, the Lady Elizabeth *daughter to King* Charles *the first.*

Take half a peck of Flower, half a pint of Rose-water, a pint of Ale yeast, a pint of Cream, boil it, a pound and a half of Butter, six Eggs (leave out the whites) four pound of Currans, one half pound of Sugar, one Nutmeg, and a little Salt, work it very well, and let it stand half an hour by the fire, and then work it again, and then make it up, and let it stand an hour and a half in the Oven; let not your Oven be too hot.

To make Paste of Apricocks.

Take your Apricocks, and pare them, and stone them, then boil them tender betwixt two dishes on a Chafing dish of coals, then being cold, lay it forth on a white sheet of paper, then take as much Sugar as it doth weigh, and boil it to a Candy height, with

as

A Queens Delight. 257

as much Rose-water and fair water as will melt the Sugar; then put the Pulp into the Sugar, and so let it boil till it be as thick as for marmalet, now and then stirring of it; then fashion it upon a Pie-plate like to half Apricocks, and the next day close the half Apricocks to the other, and when they are dry, they will be as clear as Amber, and eat much better then Apricocks it self.

To make Paste of Pippins like leaves, and some like Plums, with their Stones and Stalks in them.

Take Pippins pared and coared, and cut in pieces, and boiled tender, so strain them, and take as much Sugar as the Pulp doth weigh, and boil it to a Candy height, with as much Rose-water and fair water as will melt it, then put the Pulp into the hot Sugar, and let it boil until it be as thick as Marmalet; then fashion it on a Pie-plate, like Oaken leaves, and some like half Plums, the next day close the half Plums together; and if you please you may put the stones and stalks in them, and dry them in an Oven, and if you will have them

them look green, make the paste w[hen]
Pippins are green; and if you will ha[ve]
them look red, put a little Conserve [of]
Barberries in the Paste, and if you wil[l]
keep any of it all the year, you mu[st]
make it as thin as Tart stuff, and put i[t]
in Gallipots.

To make Paste of Elecampane roots, an ex[-]
cellent remedy for the Cough of the Lung[s.]

Take the youngest Elecampane root[s]
and boil them reasonably tender, the[n]
pith them and peel them, and so beat [them]
in a Mortar, then take twice as much s[u-]
gar as the Pulp doth weigh, and so bo[il]
it to a Candy height, with as much rose
water as will melt it; then put the Pu[lp]
into the sugar with the Pap of a ro[a]st[ed]
Apple, then let it boil till it be thic[k,]
then drop it on a Pie-plate, and so dry [it]
in an Oven till it be dry.

To make Paste of flowers of the colour [of]
Marble, tasting of natural flowers.

Take every sort of pleasing flowe[r]
as Violets, Cowslips, Gilly-flowe[rs]
Roses or Marygolds, and beat them

a Mortar, each flower by it self with sugar, till the sugar become the colour of the flower, then put a little Gum Dragon steept in water into it, and beat it into a perfect paste; and when you have half a dozen colours, every flower will take of his nature, then rowl the paste therein, and lay one piece upon another, in mingling sort, so rowl your paste in small rowls, as big and as long as your finger, then cut it off the bigness of a small nut, overthwart, and so rowl them thin, that you may see a knife through them, so dry them before the fire till they be dry.

To make Paste of Rasberries or English Currans.

Take any of the Frails, and boil them tender on a Chafing-dish of coals betwixt two dishes and strain them, with the pap of a roasted Apple, then take as much Sugar as the Pulp doth weigh, and boil to a Candy height with as much Rose-water as will melt it: then put the Pulp into the hot Sugar, and let it boil leasurely till you see it as thick as Marmalet, then fashion it on a Pie-plate, and put

put it into the Oven with two billets o wood, that the plate touch not the bottom, and so let them dry leasurely till they be dry.

To make Naples Bisket.

Take of the same stuff the Mackaroons are made of, and put to it an ounce of Pin apple-seeds in a quarter of a pound of stuff, for that is all the difference between the Mackaroons and the Naples Bisket.

To make Italian Biskets.

Take a quarter of a pound of searsed Sugar, and beat it in an Alabaster Mortar with the white of an Egg, and a little Gum Dragon steep in Rose-water, to bring it to a perfect Paste, then mould it up with a little Annifeed and a grain of Musk; then make it up like Dutch bread, and bake it on a Pye-plate in a warm Oven, till they rise somewhat high and white, take them out, but handle them not till they be throughly dry and cold.

A Queens Delight.

To make Prince Biskets.

Take a pound of searsed Sugar, and a [p]ound of fine flower, eight Eggs with [t]wo of the reddest yolks taken out, and [to] beat together one whole hour, then [ta]ke you Coffins, and indoice them over [w]ith Butter very thin, then to it put an [o]unce of Anniseeds fine dusted, and [w]hen you are ready to fill your Coffins, [p]ut in the Anniseeds, and so bake it in an [O]ven as hot as for Manchet, &c.

[T]o make Marchpane to Ice and Gild, and garnish it according to Art.

Take Almonds, and blanch them out [o]f seething water, and beat them till [t]hey come to a fine Paste in a stone Mor[t]ar, then take fine searsed Sugar, and so [b]eat it all together till it come to a per[f]ect paste, putting in now and then a [s]poonfull of Rose-water, to keep it [f]rom Oyling; then cover your March[p]ane with a sheet of paper as big as a [C]harger, then cut it round by that char[g]er, and set an edge about it as about a [T]art, then bottom it with Wafers, then [b]ake it in an Oven, or in a baking-pan,

and

and when it is hard and dry, take it out of the Oven, and Ice it with Rose-water and Sugar, and the white of an Egg, being as thick as Butter, and spread it over thin with two or three feathers, and then put it into the Oven again, and when you see it rise high and white, take it out again and garnish it with some pretty conceit, and stick some long Comfits upright in it, so gild it, then strow Biskets and Carawayes on it. If your Marchpane be oyly in beating, then put to it as much rose-water as will make it almost as thin as to Ice.

Lorenges.

Take Blossoms of flowers, and beat them in a bowl-dish, and put them in as much clarified sugar as may come to the colour of the cover, then boil them with stirring, till it is come to sugar again, then beat it fine, and searse it, and so work it up to paste with a little Gum Dragon, steep it in Rose-water, then print it with your mould, and being dry keep it up.

To make Walnuts artificial.

Take searsed sugar, and Cinnamon, of quantity alike, work it up with a little Gum Dragon, steep it in Rose-water, and print it in a mould made like a Walnut-shell, then take white sugar plates, print it in a mould made like a Walnut kernel, so when they are both dry, close them up together with a little Gum Dragon betwixt, and they will dry as they lie.

To make Collops like Bacon of Marchpane.

Take some of your Marchpane Paste, and work it in red Saunders till it be red; then rowl a broad sheet of white Paste, and the sheet of red Paste, three of the white, and four of the red, and so one upon another in mingled sorts, every red between, then cut it overthwart, till it look like Collops of Bacon, then dry it.

To make artificial Fruits.

Take a Mould made of Alablaster, three

three yolks, and tie two pieces together, and lay them in water an hour, and take as much sugar as will fill up your mould, and boil it in a *Manus Christi*, then pour it into your mould suddenly, and clap on the lid, round it about with your hand, and it will be whole and hollow, then colour it with what colour you please, half red, or half yellow, and you may yellow it with a little Saffron steept in water.

Touching Preserves and Pomanders.

To make an excellent Perfume to burn between two Rose leaves.

TAke an ounce of Juniper, an ounce of Storax, half a dozen drops o the water of Cloves, six grains o Musk, a little Gum Dragon steept in water

water, and beat all this to paste, then roll it in little pieces as big as you please, then put them betwixt two Rose leaves, and so dry them in a dish in an Oven, and being so dried, they will burn with a most pleasant smell.

To make Pomander.

Take an ounce of Benjamin, an ounce of Storax, and an ounce of Laudanum, heat a Mortar very hot, and beat all these Gums to a perfect paste; in beating of it, put in six grains of Musk, four grains of Sivet; when you have beaten all this to a fine paste with your hands with Rose-water, rowl it round betwixt your hands, and make holes in the beads, and so string them while they be hot.

To make an Ipswitch water.

Take a pound of fine white Castle Sope, shave it thin in a pint of Rose-water, and let it stand two or three dayes; then pour all the water from it, and put to it half a pint of fresh water, and so let it stand one whole day, then pour out that, and put half a pint more, and let it stand a night more, then put to it half an ounce of powder called sweet Marjoram, a quarter of an ounce of powder of wintersavory, two or three drops of the Oyl of Spike, and the Oyl of Cloves, three grains of Musk, and as much Ambergreese; work all these together in a fair Mortar, with the powder of an Almond Cake dried, and beaten as small as fine Flower, so roul it round in your hands in Rose-water.

To make a sweet Smell.

Take the Maste of a sweet Apple tree, being gathered betwixt the two Lady dayes, and put to it a quarter of Damask Rose-water, and dry it in a dish in an Oven; wet it in drying two or three times with Rose-water, then put to it an ounce of Benjamin, an ounce of Storax Calamintæ; these Gums being beaten to powder, with a few leaves of Roses, then you may put what cost of Smells you will bestow, as much Civet or Ambergreese, and beat it all together in a Pomander or a Bracelet.

Touch-

Touching VVine.

To make Hypocras.

Take four gallons of Claret Wine, eight ounces of Cinnamon, three Oranges, of Ginger, Cloves, and Nutmegs a small quantity, Sugar six pound, three sprigs of Rosemary, bruise all the spices somewhat small, and so put them into the Wine, and keep them close stopped, and often shaked together a day or two, then let it run through a gelly bag twice or thrice with a quart of new Milk.

The Lady Thornburghs Syrup of Elders.

Take Elder-berries when they be red, bruise them in a stone Mortar, strain the juyce, and boil it to a Consumption of almost half, scum it very clear, take it off the fire whilest it is hot, put in sugar to the thickness of a syrup; put it no more on the fire, when it is cold, put it into glasses, not filling them to the top, for it will work like Beer.

This cleanseth the stomach and spleen, and taketh away all obstructions of the Liver, by taking the quantity of a spoonful in a morning, and fasting a short time after it.

To make gelly of Raspis the best way.

Take the Raspis, and set them over the fire in a Posnet, and gather out the thin juyce, the bottom of the skillet being cooled with fair water, and strain it with a fine strainer, and when you have as much as you will, then weigh it with sugar, and boil them till they come to a gelly, which you may perceive by drawing your finger on the back of the spoon.

To dry Fox Skins.

Take your she Fox skins, nail them upon a board as strait as you can, then brush them as clean as you can, then take Aqua Fortis, and put into it a six pence, and still put in more as long as it will dissolve it, then wash your skin over with this water, and set it to dry in the Sun; and when it is dry, wash it over with the spirits of Wine; this must be done in hottest time of summer.

Choice Secrets made known.

To make true Magistery of Pearl.

Dissolve two or three ounces of fine seed Pearl in distilled Vinegar, and when it is perfectly dissolved, and all taken up; pour the Vinegar into a clean glass Bason; then drop some few drops of Oyl of Tartar upon it, and it will cast down

down the Pearl into fine powder, then pour the Vinegar clean off softly, then put to the Pearl clear Conduit or Spring water, pour that off, and do so often until the taste of the Vinegar and Tartar be clean gone, then dry the powder of Pearl upon warm embers, and keep it for your use.

How to make Hair grow.

Take half a pound of Aqua Mellis in the Spring time of the year, warm a little of it every morning when you rise, in a Sawcer, and tie a little sponge to a fine box comb, and dip it in the water, and therewith moisten the roots of the hair, in combing it, and it will grow long, thick, and curled in a very short time.

To write Letters of secrets that they cannot be read without the directions following

Take fine Allum, beat it small, and put a reasonable quantity of it into water, then write with the said water.

The work cannot be read, but by steeping your paper into fair running water. You

You may likewise write with Vinegar, or the juyce of Lemon or Onion, if you would read the same, you must hold it before the fire.

How to keep Wine from sowering.

Tie a piece of very salt Bacon on the inside of your barrel, so as it touch not the Wine, which will preserve Wine from sowering.

To take out spots of Grease or Oyl.

Take bones of sheeps feet, burn them almost to ashes, then bruise them to powder, and put of it on the spot, and lay it in the Sun when it shineth hottest, when the powder becomes black, lay on fresh in the place till it fetch out the spots, which will be done in a very short time.

To make hair grow black, though any color.

Take a little Aqua Fortis, put therein a groat or six pence, as to the quantity of the aforesaid water, then set both to dissolve before the fire, then dip a
small

small spunge in the said water, and wet your beard or hair therewith, but touch not the skin.

King Edwards *Perfume*.

Take twelve spoonfuls of right red Rose water, the weight of six pence in fine powder of sugar, and boil it on hot Embers and Coals softly, and the house will smell as though it were full of Roses; but you must burn the sweet Cipress wood before, to take away the gross air.

Queen Elizabeths *Perfume*.

Take eight spoonfuls of Compound water, the weight of two pence in fine powder of sugar, and boil it on hot Embers and Coals softly, and half an ounce of sweet Marjoram dried in the sun, the weight of two pence of the powder of Benjamin. This Perfume is very sweet and good for the time.

Mr. Ferene *of the* New Exchange, *Perfumer to the Queen, his rare Dentifrice so much approved of at Court.*

First take eight ounces of Irios roots, also four ounces of Pomistone, and eight ounces of Cutel bone; also eight ounces of mother of Pearl, and eight ounces of Corral, and a pound of brown sugar-candy, and a pound of Brick if you desire to make them red; but he did oftner make them white, and then instead of the Brick did take a pound of fine Alablaster; all this being throughly beaten and sifted through a fine searse, the powder is then ready prepared to make up in a paste, which must be done as follows.

To make the said powder into a Paste.

Take a little Gum Dragant, and lay it in steep twelve hours, in Orange flower water or Damask Rose-water, and when it is dissolved, take the sweet Gum, and grinde it on a Marble stone with the aforesaid powder; and mixing some crums of white bread, it will come into a Paste, the which you may make Dentifrices, of what shape or fashion you please, but long rolls is the most commodious for your use.

The Receipt of the Lady Kents powder, presented by her Ladyship to the Queen.

Take white Amber, Crabs eyes, red Corral, Harts-horn and Pearl, all prepared severall, of each a like proportion, tear and mingle them, then take Harts-horn gelly, that hath some Saffron put into a bag, dissolve into it while the gelly is warm, then let the gelly cool, and therewith make a paste of the powders, which being made up into little balls, you must dry gently by the fire side. Pearl is prepared by dissolving it with the juyce of Lemons, Amber prepared by beating it to powder; so also Crabs eyes and Corral, Harts-horn prepared by burning it in the fire, and taking the shires of it especially, the pith wholly rejected.

A Cordial Water of Sir Walter Raleigh.

Take a Gallon of Strawberries, and put them into a pint of *Aqua vitæ*, let them stand so four or five dayes, strain them gently out, and sweeten the water as you please with fine Sugar, or else with perfume.

The Lady Malets *Cordial Water*

Take a pound of fine Sugar beaten, and put to it a quart of running water, pour it three or four times through a bag; then put a pint of Damask Rose water, which you must alwayes pour still through the bag, then four penniworth of Angelica water, four pence in Clove water, four pence of Rosa solis, one pint of Cinnamon water, or three pints and half of *Aqua vitæ*, as you finde it in taste; put all these together three or four times through the bag or strainer, and then take half an ounce of good Muskallis, and cut them grosly, and put them into a glass, and fill them with the water, &c.

A Soveraign water of Dr. Stephens, *which he long time used, wherewith he did many Cures; he kept it secretly till a little before his Death, and then he gave it to the Lord Arch-Bishop of* Canterbury *in writing, being as followeth, viz.*

Take a Gallon of good Gascoine Wine,

Wine, and take Ginger, Gallingale, Cinamon, Nutmegs, Cloves, Grains, Aniseeds, Fennil-seed, of every of them a dram, then take Caraway-seed, of red Mints, Roses, Thime, Pellitory of the Wall, Rosemary, Wilde Thime, Camomil, the leaves, if you cannot get the flowers, of small Lavender, of each a handfuul, then bray the spices small, and bray the hearbs, and put all into the Wine, and let it stand so twelve hours, stirring it divers times, then still it in a Limbeck, and keep the first water, for it is best, then put the second water by it self, for it is good, but not of such vertues, &c.

The Vertue of this Water.

It comforts the Spirits Vital, and helps all inward diseases that come of cold, it is good against the shaking of the Palsey, it cures the contraction of the Sinnews, helps the conception of women if they be barren, it kills the worms in the Belly and Stomach; it cures the cold Dropsie, and helps the stone in the Bladder, and in the Reins of the Back; it helps shortly the stinking breath, and whosoever useth this water morning and evening, (and not too often) it preserveth

serveth him in good liking, and will make him seem young very long, and comforteth nature marvellously; with this water did Doctor *Stephens* preserve his life, till extream age would not let him go or stand, and he continued five years, when all the Physicians judged he could not live a year longer, nor did he use any other Medicine but this, *&c.*

A Plague water to be taken one spoonful every four hours with one sweat every time.

Take Scabious, Betony, Pimpernel, and Turmentine roots, of each a pound, steep these all night in three gallons of strong Beer, and distill them all in a Limbeck, and when you use it, take a spoonful thereof every four hours, and sweat well after it, draw two quarts of water, if your beer be strong, and mingle them both together.

Poppy Water.

Take four pound of the flower of Poppies well pickt and sifted, steep them all night in three gallons of Ale that is strong, and still it in a Limbeck, you may

may draw two quarts, the one will be strong, and the other will be small, &c.

A Water for a Consumption, or for a brain that is weak.

Take Cream (or new Milk) and Claret Wine, of each three pints, of Violet flowers, Bugloss and Borage flowers of each a spoonful, Comfrey, Knotgrass, and Plantain, of these half a handful, three or four Pome-waters sliced, a stick of Liquorish, some Pompion seeds and strings, put to this a Cock that hath been chased and beaten before he was killed, dress it as to boil and parboil it until there be no blood in it; then put them in a pot, and set them over your Limbeck, and the soft fire, draw out a pottle of water, then put your water in a Pipkin over a Charcoal fire, and boil it a while, dissolve therein six ounces of white Sugar-candy, and two penny weight of Saffron; when it is cold strain it into a glass, and let the Patient drink three or four spoonfuls three or four times a day blood-warm; your Cock must be cut into small pieces, and the bones broken, and in case the flowers and hearbs are hard to come by, a spoonfull of their stilled waters are to be used.

Another for the same.

Take a pottle of good Milk, one pint of Muscadine, half a pint of red Rose-water, a penny Manchet sliced thin, two handfuls of Raisins of the sun stoned, a quarter of a pound of fine sugar, sixteen Eggs beaten; mix all these together, then distill them in a common still with a soft fire, then let the Patient drink three or four spoonfuls at a time blood-warm, being sweetened with *Manus Christi* made with Corral and Pearl, when your things are all in the Still, strew four ounces of Cinnamon beaten, this water is good to put in broth, &c.

A good Stomach Water.

Take a quart of Aqua Composita, or Aqua vitæ (the smaller) and put into it one handful of Cowslip flowers, a good handful of Rosemary flowers, sweet Marjoram, a little Pellitory of the Wall, a little Betony and Balm, of each a little handful, Cinnamon half an ounce, Nutmegs a dram, Anniseeds, Coriander

riander seeds, Caroway seeds, Gromel seeds, Juniper berries, of each a dram, bruise the spice and seed, and put them into Aqua Composita, or *Aqua vitæ* with your hearbs together, and put into them a pound of very fine sugar, stir them well together, and put them into a glass, and let it stand in the Sun nine dayes, and stir it every day; two or three Dates, and a little race of Ginger sliced into it will make it the better, especially against winde, *&c.*

A Bag of Purging Ale.

Take of Agrimony, Speedwel, Liverwort, Scurvy grass, Water Cresses of each a handful, of Monk, of Rhubarb and red Madder, of each half a pound, of Horse Radishes three ounces, Liquorish two ounces, Sassafrage four ounces, Sena seven ounces, sweet Fennil-seeds two drams, Nutmegs four: pick and wash your hearbs and roots, and bruise them all in a Mortar, and put them in a bag made of a Bolter, and so hang them in three galons of middle ale, and let it work in the ale, and after three dayes you may drink of it as you see occasion, *&c.*

The Ale of Health and Strength, by Vicount St. Albans.

Take Saſſafras wood half an ounce, Sarſaparilla three ounces, white Saunders one ouncce, Chamapition an ounce, China root half an ounce, Mace a quarter of an ounce, Chamapition an ounce, cut the wood as thin as may be with a knife into small pieces, and bruiſe them in a Mortar; put to them theſe ſorts of hearbs, (*viz.*) Cowſlip flowers, Roman Wormwood, of each a handfull, of Sage, Roſemary, Betony, Mugwort, Balm and ſweet Marjoram, of each half a handful, of Hops; boil all theſe in ſix gallons of Ale till it come to four, then put the wood and hearbs into ſix gallons of Ale of the ſecond wort, and boil it till it come to four, let it run from the dregs, and put your Ale together, and tun it as you do other purging Ale, &c.

A water excellent good againſt the Plague.

Take three pints of Malmſey, or Muſcadine, of Sage and Rue of each one

one handful, boil them together gen[t]ly to one pint, then strain it and set i[t] on the fire again, and put to it one pe[n]niworth of Long Pepper, Ginger fou[r] drams, Nutmegs two drams, all beate[n] together, then let it boil a little, tak[e] it off the fire, and while it is very ho[t] dissolve therein six penniworth of Mith[ridate, and three penniworth of Ve[nice Treacle, and when it is almost col[d] put to it a pint of strong Angelica w[a]ter, or so much *Aqua vitæ*, and so kee[p] it in a glass close stopped.

A cordial Cherry water.

Take a pottle of *Aqua vitæ*, tw[o] ounces of ripe Cherries stoned, Suga[r] one pound, twenty four Cloves, on[e] stick of Cinnamon, three spoonfuls of A[ni]seeds bruised, let these stand in the A[qua vitæ fifteen dayes, and when the w[a]ter hath fully drawn out the Tinctur[e] pour it off into another glass for yo[ur] use, which keep close stopped, the sp[ice] and the Cherries you may keep, for th[ey] are very good for wind in the Stomach[.]

T

The Lord Spencers Cherry water.

Take a pottle of new Sack, four pound of through ripe Cherries stoned, put them into an earthen pot, to which put an ounce of Cinnamon, Saffron unbruised one dram, tops of Balm, Rosemary or their flowers, of each one handful, let them stand close covered twenty four hours, now and then stirring them: then put them into a cold Still, to which put of beaten Amber two drams, Coriander seed one ounce, Alkermis one dram, and distill it leasurely, and when it is fully distilled, put to it twenty grains of Musk. This is an excellent Cordiall, good for Faintings and Swoundings, for the Crudities of the Stomach, Winde and swelling of the Bowels, and divers other evil Symptomes in the body of Men and Women.

The hearbs to be distilled for Usquebath.

Take Agrimony, Fumitory, Betony, Bugloss, Wormwood, Harts-tongue, Carduus Benedictus, Rosemary, Angelica,

lica, Tormentil, of each of these fo[ur?]
every gallon of Ale one handfull, An[ise]
seeds and Liquorice well bruised half [a]
pound. Still all these together, an[d]
when it is stilled, you must infuse Cina[-]
mon, Nutmeg, Mace, Liquorice, Date[s]
and Raisins of the Sun, and Sugar wha[t]
quantity you please. The infusion mu[st]
be till the colour please you.

Dr. Kings way to make Mead.

Take five quarts and a pint of Wate[r]
and warm it, then put one quart of Ho[-]
ney to every gallon of Liquor, one Li[-]
mon, and a quarter of an ounce of Nu[t-]
megs; it must boil till the scum ri[se]
black, that you will have it quick[ly]
ready to drink, squeeze into it a Lem[on]
when you tun it. It must be cold befo[re]
you tun it up.

To make Syrup of Rasberries.

Take nine quarts of Rasberries, cle[an]
pickt, and gathered in a dry day, a[nd]
put to them four quarts of good Sac[k]
into an earthen pot, then paste it up v[e-]
ry close, and set it in a Cellar for t[en]
day[s]

dayes, then distill it in a Glass or Rose-still, then take more Sack and put in Rasberries to it, then when it hath taken out all the colour of the Raspiss, strain it out, and put in some fine Sugar to your taste, and set it on the fire, keeping it continually stirring till the scum doth rise, then take it off the fire, let it not boil, skim it very clean, and when it is cold put it to your distilled Raspis, but colour it no more then to make it a pale Claret wine. This put into bottles or glasses stopt very close.

To make Lemon Water.

Take twelve of the fairest Lemons, slice them, and put them into two pints of White wine, and put to them Cinamon two drams, Gallingale two drams; of Rose leave, Borage and Bugloss flowers of each one handfull, of yellow Saunders one dram; steep all these together twelve hours, then distill them gently in a Glass Still untill you have distilled one pint and an half of the water, and then adde to it three ounces of Sugar, one grain of Ambergreese, and you will have a most pleasing

sing cleansing Cordial water for man uses.

To make Gilly-flower Wine.

Take two ounces of dried Gilly-flowers, and put them into a pottle of Sack, and beat three ounces of Sugar-candy, or fine Sugar, and grinde some Ambergreese, and put it in the bottle and shake it oft, then run it through a gelly bag, and give it for a great Cordial after a weeks standing or more. You make Lavender Wine as you do this.

The Lady Spotswoods Stomach Water.

Take white Wine one pottle, Rosemary and Cowslip flowers, of each one handful, as much Betony leaves, Cinnamon and Cloves grosly beaten, of both one ounce; steep all these three days stirring it often; then put to it Mithridate four ounces, and stir it together, and distill it in an ordinary still.

Water of Time for the passion of the Heart.

Take a quart of white Wine, and a pint of Sack, steep in it as much Broad Thime as it will wet, put to it of Galingale and Calamus Aromaticus, of each one ounce, Cloves, Mace, Ginger, and grains of Paradise two drams, step these all night, the next morning distill it in an ordinary Still, drink it warm with Sugar.

A Receipt to make Damnable Hum.

Take species de Gemmis, Aromaticum Rosatum, Diarhodon Abbatis, Lætificans Galeni, of each four drams, Loaf sugar beaten to powder half a pound, small *Aqua vitæ* three pints, strong Angelica water one pint; mix all these together, and when you have drunk it to the dregs, you may fill it up again with the same quantity of waters. The same powders will serve twice, and after twice using it, it must be made new again.

An admirable Water for sore Eyes.

Take *Lapis Tutiæ*, Aloes, Hepatica, fine hard Sugar, of each three drams, beat them very small, and put them into a Glass of three pints, to which put red Rose water and white Wine, of each one pint; set the Glass in the Sun in the moneth of *July*, for the whole moneth, shaking it twice in a day for all that while; then use it as followeth, put one drop thereof into the Eye in the evening, when the party is in bed, and one drop in the morning an hour before the patient riseth: Continue the use of it till the Eyes be well. The older the Water, the better it is. Most approved.

A Snail Water for weak Children, and Old people.

Take a pottle of Snails, and wash them well in two or three waters, and then in small Beer, bruise them shell and all, then put them into a gallon of red Cowes milk, red Rose leaves dried the whites cut off, Rosemary, sweet Marjoram

Marjoram, of each one handful, and so distill them in a cold still, and let it drop upon powder of white Sugarcandy in the receiver; drink of it first and last, and at four a clock in the afternoon, a Wine glass full at a time.

Clary water for the Back, Stomach, &c.

Take three gallons of midling Beer, put it in a great brasse Pot of four gallons, and put to it ten handfuls of Clary gathered in a dry day, Raysins of the Sun stoned three Pounds, Anniseeds and Liquorish of each four ounces, the whites and shells of tweny four Eggs, or half so many if there be not so much need in the back, the shells small, and mix them, with the whites; put to the bottoms of three whites loaves, put into the receiver one und of white Sugarcandy, or so much e loaf sugar beaten small, and distill t through a Limbeck, keep it close, and seldom without it, for it reviveth ve. much the stomach and heart, strength- h the Back, procureth Appetite nd digestion, driveth away Melancholy, dness and heaviness of the Heart, &c.

Dr. Montfords *Cordial Water*.

Take Angelica leaves twelve handfuls, six leaves of Carduus Benedictus, Balm and Sage, of each five handfuls, the seeds of Angelica and sweet Fennil, of each five ounces bruised, scraped and bruised Liquorish twelve ounces, Aromaticum Rosatum, Diamoscus dulcis, of each six drams; the hearbs being cut small, the seeds and Liquorish bruised, infuse them into two gallons of Canary Sack for twenty four hours, then distill it with a gentle fire, and draw off onely five pints of the spirits, which mix with one pound of the best Sugar dissolved into a syrup in half a pint of pure red Rose-water.

Aqua mirabilis, Sir Kenelm Digby's way.

Take Cubebs, Gallingale, Cardamus, Mellilot flowers, Cloves, Mace, Ginger, Cinnamon, of each one dram bruised small, juyce of Celandine o pint, juyce of Spearmint half a pint, juyce of Balm half a pint, Sugar o pound, flower of Cowslips, Rosemary, Bora

Borage, Buglosse, Marigolds, of each two drams, the best Sack three pints, strong Angelica water one pint, red Rose-water half a pint, bruise the spices and flowers, and steep them in the Sack and juyces one night, the next morning distill it in an ordinary or glass still, and first lay Harts tongue leaves in the bottom of the still.

The Vertues of the precedent Water.

This water preserveth the Lungs without grievances, and helpeth them; being wounded, it suffereth not the blood to putrefie, but multiplieth the same; this water suffereth not the heart to burn, nor melancholy, nor the spleen to be lifted up above nature, it expelleth the Rhume, preserveth the Stomach, conserveth Youth, and procureth a good colour, it preserveth Memory, it destroyeth the Palsie; if this be given to one a dying, a spoonful of it reviveth him; in the summer use one spoonful a week fasting, in the winter two spoonfuls.

A Water for fainting of the Heart.

Take Bugloss and red Rose-water,

of each one pint, Milk half a pint, Anniseeds and Cinnamon grosly bruised, of each half an ounce, Maiden-hair two handfuls, Harts tongue one handful, both shred, mix all together, and distill it in an ordinary still, drink of it morning and evening with a little sugar.

A Surfeit Water.

Take half a bushel of red Corn Poppy, put it into a large dish, cover it with brown paper, and lay another dish upon it, let it in an Oven after brown bread is baked divers times till it be dry, which put into a pottle of good *Aqua vitæ*, to which put Raisins of the sun stoned half a pound, six figs sliced, three Nutmegs sliced, two flakes of Mace bruised, two races of Ginger sliced, one stick of Cinnamon bruised, Liquorish sliced one ounce, Anniseed Fennil-seed, and Cardamums bruised, of each one dram; put all these into a broad glass body, and lay first some Poppy in the bottom; then some of the other Ingredients, then Poppy again, and so till the glass be full;
then

then put in the *Aqua vitæ*, and let it infuse till it be strong of the spices, and very red with the Poppy, close covered, of the which take two or three spoonfuls upon a Surfeit, and when all the liquor is spent, put more *Aqua vitæ* to it, and it will have the same effect the second time, but no more after.

D. Butlers *Cordial Water against Melancholly, &c. Most approved.*

Take the flowers of Cowslips, Marigolds, Pinks, Clove-gilly-flowers, single stock Gilly-flowers, of each four handfuls, the flowers of Rosemary, and Damask Roses, of each three handfuls, Borage, and Bugloss flowers, and Balm leaves, of each two handfuls; put them in a quart of Canary Wine into a great bottle or jugg close stopped with a cork, sometimes stirring the flowers and wine together, adding to them Anniseeds bruised one dram, two Nutmegs sliced, English Saffron two penniworth; after some time infusion, distill them in a cold Still with a hot fire, hanging at the Nose of the Still,

Ambergreese and Musk, of each one grain: then to the distilled water put white Sugarcandy finely beaten six ounces, and put the glass, wherein they are into hot water for one hour. Take of this water at one time three spoonfuls thrice a week, or when your are ill, it cureth all melancholy fumes, and infinitely comforts the spirits.

The admirable and most famous Snail water.

Take a peck of garden shell Snails, wash them well in small Beer, and put them in an hot Oven, till they have done making a noise, then take them out, and wipe them well from the green froth that [is] upon them, and bruise them shells an[d] all in a stone Mortar, then take a qua[rt] of earth Worms, scower them with Sal[t] slit them and wash them well with w[a]ter from their filth, and in a stone Mo[r]tar beat them to pieces, then lay [in] the bottom of your distilled pot A[n]gelica two handfuls, and two handf[uls] of Celandine upon them, to which p[ut] two quarts of Rosemary flowers, Be[ars] foot, Agrimony, red Dock roo[t] Ba[lm]

...rk of Barberries, Betony, wood Sor-
...l, of each two handfuls, Rue one hand-
...l; then lay the Snails and Worms on
...e top of the hearbs and flowers, then
...our on three Gallons of the strongest
...le, and let it stand all night, in the mor-
...ing put in three ounces of Cloves bea-
...n, six penniworth of beaten Saffron,
...d on the top of them six ounces of
...aved Harts-horn, then set on the Lim-
...eck, and close it with paste, and so re-
...ive the water by pints, which will be
...ne in all, the first is the strongest, where-
...f take in the morning two spoonfuls in
...ur spoonfuls of small Beer, and the like
...the afternoon; you must keep a good
...et, and use moderate exercise to warm
...e blood.

This water is good against all ob-
...uctions whatsoever. It cureth a Con-
...mption and Dropsie, the stopping of
...e Stomach and Liver. It may be di-
...lled with Milk for weak people and
...ildren with Harts-tongue and Elecam-
...ne.

P 4

A singular Mint Water.

Take a still full of Mints, put Balm and Penniroyal, of each one good handful, steep them in Sack, or Lees of Sack twenty four hours, stop it close, and stir it now and then: Distill it in an ordinary Still with a very quick fire, and keep the Still with wet clothes, put into the Receiver as much sugar as will sweeten it, and so double distill it.

Distillings.

A most excellent Aqua Celestis taught Mr. Philips Apothecary.

TAke of Cinnamon one dram, Ginger half a dram, the three sorts Saunders, of each of them three quarters of an ounce, Mace and Cubebs of each them one dram, Cardamon the biggest and lesser, of each three drams, Setwell roots half an ounce, Anniseed, Fennil-seed, Basil-seed, of each two drams, Angelica roots, Gilly flowers, Thime, Calimint, Liquorish, Casamus Masterwort, Penniroyal, Mint, Mother of Thime, Marjoram, of each two drams, red Rose-seed, the flowers of Sage and Betony, of each a dram and a half, Cloves Galingal, Nutmegs, of each two drams, the flowers of Stechados, Rosemary, Borage, and Bugloss flowers, of each a dram and half, Citron rindes three drams; bruise them all, and put in these Cordial powders, Diamber Aromaticum, Diamuscum, Diachoden, the spices made with Pearl, of each three drams; infuse all these in twelve pints of *Aqua vitæ*, in a glass close stopped for fifteen dayes, often shaking it, then let it be put in a Limbeck close stopped, and let it be distilled gently; when you have done, hang it in a cloth, two drams of Musk, half a dram of Ambergreese, and ten or twelve grains of gold, and so receive it to your use.

Hypocras taught by Dr. Twine for winde in the Stomach.

Take Pepper, Grains, Ginger, of each half an ounce, Cinnamon, Cloves, Nutmegs, Mace, of each one ounce grosly beaten, Rosemary, Agrimony, both shred, of each a few crops, red rose leaves a pretty quantity, as an indifferent gripe, a pound of Sugar beaten, lay these to steep in a gallon of good Rhennish or White Wine in a close vessel, stirring it two or three times a day the space of three or four dayes together, then strain it through an Hypocras strainer, and drink a draught of it before meat half an hour, and sometimes after to help digestion.

Marigold flowers distilled, good for the pain of the Head.

Take Marigold flowers, and distil them, then take a fine cloth and wet it the aforesaid distilled water, and so lay it to the forehead of the Patient, and being so applied, let him sleep if he can: this with Gods help will cease the pain.

A water good for Sun-burning.

Take water drawn off the Vine dropping, the flowers of white Thorn, Bean flowers, Water Lilly-flowers, Garden Lilly-flowers, Elder-flowers, and Tansie flowers, Althea flowers, the whites of Eggs, French Barley.

The Lady Giffords Cordial water.

Take four quarts of *Aqua vitæ*, Borrage and Poppy water, of each a pint, two pound of Sugarcandy, one pound of Figs sliced, one pound of Raisins of the Sun stoned, two handfuls of red Roses clipped and dried, one handful of red Mint, half a handful of Rosemary, as much of Hysop, a few Cloves; put all these in a great double Glass close stopped, and set it in the Sun three moneths, and so use it.

A Water for one pensive and very sick, to comfort the heart very excellent.

Take a good spoonful of Manus Christi beaten very small into powder, then take a quarter of a pound of very fine sugar, and beat it small, and six spoonfuls of Cinnamon water, and put to it, and ten spoonfuls of red Rose water, mingle all these together, and put them in a dish, and set them over a soft fire five or six walms, and so let it be put into a glass, and let the party drink thereof a spoonful or two as he shall see cause.

To perfume Water.

Take Malmsey or any kinde of sweet water, then take Lavander, Spike, sweet Marjoram, Balm, Orange peels, Thime, Basil, Cloves, Bay leaves, Woodbine flowers, red and white Roses, and still them all together.

FINIS.

THE TABLE.

A.

Aches to take away   38, 41, 72, 108,
110, 153, 156, 157, 184
Abortion to prevent   121
After-birth to bring away   159, 160
Ague of all sorts to cure   16, 32, 52, 57,
127, 161
Ague in womens breast   110, 167
Ale to purge most excellent   2, 280, 281
Ambergreese tincture to make, and use 24
Amber pills for a Consumption   3
Appetite to help   50, 61, 184
Appoplex to cure   236
Aqua mirabilis to make   290
Almond milk to make   82, 83, 108

B.

Biting of a snake   154
Backs heat to cool   94, 95
Back to strengthen 66, 135, 184, 191, 289
Balsam most excellent, with its use   95,
123, 125
Belly-ake to cure   184
Belly hard to dissolve   155
Biles and Botches to cure 81, 89, 112, 152,
188.   *Blood*

Barly-water or ptisan, one sort. p. 128

The Table.

Bloud to cleanse   10,148,161
Biting of a mad Dog   41,152,154
Bloudy flux to help 42,106,108,130,184
Bleeding at Nose to stanch   163
Bladder to cleanse   169,237
Bones out of joynt to set   104,153,189
Breaths shortness to remedy   5
Breath stinking to cure   53,111,196,276
Brain to strengthen   17,86,178,196,236
Burning to help   60,77,78,95,104,125, 149,162,189
Breasts sore to cure   85,90,91,109,110, 117,147
Bruises to cure. 36,38,90.104,122,125, 144,156,184,188
Bursten to remedy   145
Balsam Luccatelloes to make, and its virtues   179
Bag restorative for the stomach   57

C.

Canker to cure   36,41,152
Cock water   14
Cancer to prevent and cure   36,108,135
China broth in a Consumption   34
Choler to purge   49,102,176,177,233
Childe to bring again when born   159,160
Consumption to cure   3,9,10,14,27,34, 42,123,186,299,278,279,295
Cold to help   27,88,164,206
                              Cough

The Table.

Cough to take away   55, 56, 59, 62, 63, 100, 164
Conception to help   88, 168, 184, 235, 276
Costiveness to remove   159
Cholick to cure   44, 63, 96, 99, 105, 125, 166, 170
Corns to take away   104, 146
Cramp to cure   141
Cordials most excellent   7, 14, 274, 275, 285, 290
Cordial water   2
Conserves of all sorts to make, and their vertues   234, 235, 236
Mrs. Chaunce her Purge   165
Cordial waters for the sick   14

D.

Drink for the Scurvy   149
Diet Drink for a Fistula   70
Diet Drink for one that hath no speech in sickness   71
Deafness to help   45, 105, 162
Dead flesh to prevent   152
Digestion to procure, 6, 15, 30, 125, 196, 244
Dropsie to cure, 11, 16, 42, 52, 64, 276, 295
Diseases cured without taking any thing at the mouth   49
Drink for Rhume and Phlegm   57
Drink for a hot Feaver   98, 128
Drink to keep the mouth moist   132

Electuary

The Table.

E.

Electuary for the stomach
Electuary for the poison of the heart, 9
Eyes sore to cure 28,147,148,189,28
Eyes full of Rhume 18,32,110,18
Eyes weak to strengthen 130,18
Eyes having a Pin or Web 171,17
Eyes redness to take away 171,173,18

F.

Face sweld to asswage 1
Faces redness and pimples to cure 41
53,54,55,173,18
Face bruised 14
Face fair to make 115,18
Faintness to take away 86,133,283,29
Falling sickness to cure 49,88,142,23
Feavers all sorts to remove 2,12 25,6
98,128,13
Festers in the flesh to cure 4
Fellons to cure 41,48,102,18
Fire to take out 18
Fistula to cure 70,79,117,15
Finger sore to heal 8
Flux or Looseness to stay 1
Freckles to take away 14
Fish to take by angling 10

G.

Gascony Powder to make 18
Gout to cure 42,50,77,88,140,1
Gold

The Table.

Golden colour without gold to make	114
Green sickness to cure	69,85
Gravel to cleanse	185
Glisters for a hot Feaver	132
Glisters for the Winde	30,160

H.

Hair to grow thick	100,270
Hair to take away	55
Hardness to dissolve	189
Heart to chear	52,87,235
Heads lightness in sickness	72
Head-ache to cure	41,96,120,125,235
Heads breaking out in Children	148
Hearts passion to take away	98,287
Heart-burn to cure	291
Hearing	45
Hearbs boild in Broth	65,166
Humors watery to purge	102,184
Humors hot to cool	177

I.

Jaundies black and yellow to cure	16,73, 74,105
Impostumes to cure,	42,89,112,152,184
Inflammations to prevent	189
Joynts to heat	188
Iron to keep from rust	113
Itch to cure. 42,	32,77
Juyce of Liquorish to make	307
Julip for a Feaver	61

Kidneys

The Table.

K.
Kidneys ulceration to cure   5
Kidney swoln to take away   5
Kidneys to cool and cleanse   83
Kings Evil to cure   117

L.
Labor in women to help   86, 119, 130
Letters of secrets how to write   270
Letters of gold to make without gold   114
Letters of silver to make without silver ib.
Liver to strengthen and cool   17, 68, 92, 93, 184, 268, 295
Looseness to help   80, 143
Lungs to cleanse   44, 47, 59, 62, 291
Lumly's drink for a Consumption   123

M.
Mangy in a dog to cure   120
Mead to make   284
Measles to cure   29, 107, 236
Melancholy to suppress   4, 23, 52, 164, 165, 177, 291, 293
Memory to preserve   291
Megrum to cure   119
Milk in women to increase   35, 143
Milk to dry up   174
Miscarriage in women to prevent   46, 121
Mothers rising to prevent   20, 63
Mouth to keep moist   132
Morphew to take away   146

Navels

The Table.

N.

Navels coming out to help   109
Nipple to skin when raw   174, 175
Nipple to make when none   175
Noses shining to cure   53
Noses redness to cure   54
Noli me tangere   52

O.

Obstructions   10, 68, 236, 268, 295
Ointment for a hard belly   155
Oyl of Excester to make   75, 156
Oyl of Mustard-seed, and its use   77
Oyl of Eggs   75
Oyl for a shining nose   54
Oyl of Fennel, and its use   77
Oyl of Rue to make, and its use   ibid.
Oyl of Cammomil to make, and use   ibib.
Oyl of St. Johns-wort to make   131, 190
Oyl of Swallows to make   182
Oyntment green to make   36, 97, 117, 158
Oyntments and their uses   189
Oximel Compositum to make   67

P.

Palsie to cure   6, 16, 42, 52, 77, 88, 276, 291
Paracelsus Plaister to make, and vertues   150, 152
Plaister called Leaden plaister to make, and use   188, 183, 184

Plaister

The Table.

Plaister for the stomach   12
Pains to asswage   153,18
Plegme to void, 44,49,52,57,68,102,14
Plague to prevent and cure 2,9,12,17,24
    25,30,31,33,39,40,67,78,106
       107,125,142,277,28
Piles to cure   36,42,43,101,18
Powder of the Lady Kents   187,27
Powder most excellent to make   19,7
Small pox, excellent remedies 2,12,29.10
   And to prevent pitting   135,136,137
      138,139,14
   And to prevent infection   14
Pricking with a needle or thorn   10
Purge for a quartain Ague   16
Purging Ale
Purge for Children or old men   5
Pimples in the face   5
Pomatum to make   31
Purging drink most excellent   6
Purge of Dr. Mayherne   18
Purples to cure   8
Pushes to break and heal,   18
Pain in the stomach   12
Pills for a Consumption

R.

R*eins to purge*   68,88,237,27
   Rest to procure   23
Rhume to stay   32,47,57,58,100,29
       Ricke

The Table.

Rickets to cure	126, 127
Rupture to cure	129
Running of the Reins to cure	184
Restorative broth	42

S.

Saffron water to make	18
Scabs to dry up	42
Sciatica to cure	101, 156
Salve the chiefest, and its vertues	41
Scurvy to cure	149, 185
Scalding to cure	60, 77, 78, 95, 104, 125, 149, 162
Shingles to cure	153
Sinews to strengthen	86, 88, 95, 152, 189, 276
Stinging of an Adder or Wasp	154
Stepkins water for the Eyes	18
Syrup of Ale for the Whites	95
Syrup for swounding and the Brain	86
Syrup of Cordinal	10
Syrup for a Cold	27
Syrup of Turneps to make, and use	9, 19
Syrup of Citron peels to make	9, 28
Syrup of Pearmains to make	23
Syrup of Lemons to make	28
Syrup of Hysop to make	206
Syrup of Gilly-flowers	205
Skin to bring	189
Silver letters without silver to make	114

Serpents

The Table.

Serpents bitings to cure　　　　　1[?]
Sleep to procure　　　　　60, 1[?]
Snail water to make, and its vertues 2[?]
Spitting of blood to remedy　　　23
Sprains to cure　　　　　　　　1[?]
Speech in sickness to move　　71, [?]
Splinters and thorns to draw forth
Spirits to revive　　　18, 88, 276, 2[?]
Spleen distempers to rectifie　16, 41, 6[?]
　　68, 123, 164, 165, 236, 268, 2[?]
Sounding fits to cure　20, 86, 133, 2[?]
Sounding fits after Childe-birth　1
Sores of all sorts to cure 111, 117, 152, 1[?]
Stopping of the Stomach　5, 49, 63, 1[?]
　　161, 235, 236, 2[?]
Stomach cold to warm　　　15, 17[?]
Stomach hot to cool　　　　　　2
Stomach weak to strengthen　20, 57, 1[?]
　　128, 179, 283, 286, 2[?]
Stone in the Kidnies to cure　　7, 8[?]
Spirit of Castorcum
Stone in the Bladder　8, 21, 33, 45,
　　50, 52, 59, 84, 88, 94, 163, 1[?]
　　168, 170, 185, 191, [?]
Stone in the Kidneys
Strangury to help　　　　　168,
Strains to remedy
Stitches to cure　　　65, 96, 112, [?]
Sweating to prevent
　　　　　　　　　　　　　Sw

The Table.

Sweating to provoke	67
Swallow to help	51
Swelling to swage	36, 42, 104, 108, 157, 184, 188, 189
Surfeits to cure	107, 125, 292

T

Taste to restore	61
Terrils Salve	40
Tetter to cure	22, 174
Tearms to provoke	184
Teeth to make come without pain	47
Teeth to preserve	192
Tooth-ach to cure	88, 192
Thorns to draw out	41
Throws after birth to ease	118
Thrush in the mouth to remedy	36
Throat sore to cure, 51.	44, 233
Tumors to allay	42
Tissick to help	77
Tympany to remedy	65
Tincture of Ambergreese	24

U

Venom to drive from the heart	2
Ulcers to fill with flesh	189
Vomiting to stay	133
Urine sharp to cure	162
Urine to provoke	68, 99
Uvula to draw up	52
Vomit for an Ague	57
	Water

The Table.

W

Water for an Ague   16
Water to hold   91
Water very precious   18, 27
Dr. Stephens his water   18, 21
Whites and heat in the back.   94, 95
Water Cordial   8
Wormwood Cakes   15
Water of Life.   16
Warts to take away   145
Wen to cure   144
Winde to expel   30, 35, 77, 86, 122, 125, 160, 196, 282, 283
Worms to kill and avoid   16, 40, 76, 88, 89, 116, 123, 176, 276
Wounds to heal   38, 41, 90, 95, 103, 112, 115, 122, 125, 131, 152, 163, 179, 181, 188, 189, 36, 42
Wrench to cure   18
VVomen with childe to preserve them from Abortion.   121
VVoman in labour a medicine for safe deliverance   86

Y

Youth to preserve   88, 279, 291

FINIS.

The Table to the QUEENS DELIGHT.

A.

Apricocks to preserve when they are green   Page 204
Apricocks to preserve when they are ripe   203
Apricocks to dry   210, 232
Apricock Cakes   213
Apricocks to make of them Jumbals   222
Artichokes to preserve   201
Almond Bisket to make   208
Ale purging a bag   280
Ale strengthning and healthful by Sir J. Bacon   281
Aqua Mirabilis Sir Kenelm Digby's way   290
Aqua Mirabilis the vertues   291
Ambergreese the tincture   216

B.

Barberries the best way to preserve them   220

The Table.

C.

Cherries to preserve them bigger then they grow naturally 228
Cherries the ordinary way of preserving them 245
Cherries to preserve them with a quarter of their weight in Sugar 217
Cakes to make 255
Cakes to make after the maner of the Princess, the Lady Elizabeth daughter to King Charles the first. 257
Cakes of Plums 258
Cakes of Rasberries 252
Cakes of Sugar to make 250
Collops to make, like Bacon, of Marchpane 263
Clove-gilly-flowers to make a Syrup of them 205
Conserve for a Cough, or a Consumption 199
Conserve for any fruits 200
Conserve of Roses boild 209
Conserve of Roses unboild 210
Conserve of Red Roses after the Italian manner. with the vertues. 231
Conserve of Violets after the Italian manner, with the vertues 233

Conserve

The Table.

Conserve of *Borage* after the *Italian* manner, with the vertues — 234
Conserve of *Rosemary* after the *Italian* manner, with the vertues — 234
Conserve of *Betony* after the *Italian* manner with the vertues — 235
Conserve of *Sage* — 235
Conserve of the *Flowers of Lavander* — 236
Conserve of *Marjorm*, with the vertues — 236
Conserve of *Piony* after the *Italian* manner, with the vertues — 237
Candy *Cherries* — 241
Candy *Cherries* the *Italian* way — 244
Candy *Oranges* — 241
Candy *Orange Roots* — 242
Candy *Orange Peels* after the *Italian* manner, with the vertues — 243
Candy *Lemons* — 241
Candy *Citrons* — 241
Candy *Citrons* after the *Spanish* way — 243
Candy *Rosemary flowers* in the *Sun* — 237
Candy *Pippins* — 239
Candy *Pears* — 239
Candy *Apricocks* — 239
Candy *Plums* — 239
Candy *Rockandy flowers* — 239
Candy *Spanish flowers* — 240
Candy *Grapes* — 241

The Table.

Candy Barberries 24
Candy Suckets 24
Candy Angelica 24
Candy Chycory roots after the Italian manner, with the vertues 24

D.

Damsins to preserve them 229, 29
Dentifrice by Mr. Ferene of the New Exchange, Perfumer to the Queen, highly approved of at the Court. 27
Distilled Marigold flowers 29

E.

Elecampane to preserve 20

F.

Fruits to preserve green 19
Fruits to dry after they are preserved to candy them 20
Fruits artificial 20
Fox Skins to dry 20
French tart to make 2

G.

Grapes to preserve 196, 20
Hypocr.

The Table.

H.

Hypocras made by Dr. Twine for the winde in the Stomach. 298
Hair to make it grow 270
Hair to make it black, though of any other colour. 271

I.

Italian Bisket to make 260
Jelly of Pippins to make 218
Jelly of Raspis to make 268
Ipswich balls to make 265
Juyce of Liquorish to make 207

K.

Countess of Kent's Powder, the true Receipt of it as she presented it to the Queen for her private use 274

L.

Lemons to preserve 199
Letters so to write them, that they cannot be read without the directions 270
Lozenges to make of red Roses 220, 262

The Table.

M.

Marchpane to Ice and Gild, and garnish it according to Art   261
Magistery of Pearl to make it   269
Mead of Dr. Kings making   234
Marigold flowers distilled   298
Marmalet of Damsins   245
Marmalet of Oranges   247, 249
Marmalet of Orange Cakes   249
Marmalet of tender Plums   246
Marmalet of Quinces   ibid

N.

Naples Bisket to make   260

O.

Oranges to preserve the French way   224
Orange and Lemons to preserve   199
Orange Cakes   261

P.

Pear-plums green to preserve them   204

Pear-

The Table.

Pear-plums to preserve them when they are ripe. 203
Plums black or red to preserve 229
Plums green to preserve 225
Plums to dry them 228, 231
Pears to dry without Sugar, and otherwise. 205, 229, 230
Pippins to preserve them 198
Pippins to preserve them when they are green 204
Pippins to preserve them when they are ripe 203
Pippins to dry them 229, 230
Pippins to dry them without Sugar. 205
Pippins to make a Gelly of them 218
Peaches to preserve when they are green 204
Peaches to preserve when they are ripe 203
Pomatum to make 212
Prince Bisket to make 261
Powder Sweet the best way to break it 211
Powder of the Countess of Kent, the truest Receipt of it, as she presented it to the Queen for her private use 274
Perfume of King Edward the Sixth 272
Perfume of Queen Elizabeth 272
Perfume to make 212

Per-

The Table.

Perfume for cloth and gloves — 2
Perfume to burn it betwixt two Rose leaves — 264
Perfume water to make it — 300
Pomanders to make — 265
Paste of Oranges and Lemons — 251
Paste of Genoa Citrons — 253
Paste of Apricocks — 256
Paste of Pippins like Leaves, and some like Plums with their Stones and Stalks in them — 257
Paste of Elecampane roots — 258
Paste of flowers of the colour of Marmalet, tasting of natural flowers — 258
Paste of Rasberries and English Currans — 259

Q.

Quinces to preserve them white — 19
Quinces to preserve them white or red — 20
Quinces to order them for Pies — 21
Quinces to make Chips of them — 22
Quinces to make Jumbals of them — 22
Quiddony of Pippins, of Ruby, or any other Amber colour — 24
Quiddony of all kindes of Plums — 24

The Table.

R.

REspass to preserve 197
Receipt for to make damnable Hum 287

S.

SWeet Smell 267
Spots of grease or oyl to take them out 271
Sugar cakes to make 250
Sugar of Wine to make 221
Sugar of Wormwood to make 221
Sugar of Annifeeds to make 221
Sugar of Roses to make 298
Syrup of Clove-gilly-flowers 205
Syrup of Hysop water 206
Syrup of Lemons 221
Syrup of Citrons 221
Syrup of Elders by the Lady Thornburgh 267
Syrup of Rasberries 284

U.

Vsquebath the best way to make it 217
Vsquebath, Hearbs to be distilled for it 283

Wine

The Table.

W.

Wine of Raysins to make 214
Wine of Rasberries to make 215
Wine of Gilly-flowers to make 286
Wine of Hypocras 167
Wine to keep it from sowering 171
Walnuts to preserve them 201
Walnuts artificial to make them 263
Water by the Lady Spotswood 286
Water cordial by the Lady Mallet 275
Water of Cherries by the Lady Spencer 283
Water by the Lady Gifford 299
Aqua mirabilis by Sir Kenelm Digby 290
Aqua Celestis by Mr. Philips, Apothecary 296
Water Cordial against Melancholly by D. Butler 293
Water Cordial by Dr. Mumford 290
Water Cordial by Sir Walter Raleigh 274
Water of a most Soveraign use made by D. Stephens, which a little before his death he presented to the Arch-Bishop of Canterbury, the vertues of it 275, 276
Water for the Eyes. 288
Water for weak Children 288

VVa-

The Table.

Water for a weak back and stomach   289
Water for the Plague   277, 281
Water for pensive and very sick persons   300
Water for a Consumption or weak Brain   278, 279
Water for the stomach   279
Water for Sun-burning   299
Water for a Surfeit   292
Water for the swimming of the heart   291
Water of Time for the passion of the Heart   287
Water of Cherries   282
Water Cordial of Cherries   282
Water of Lemons   285
Water of Oranges   206
Water perfumed   300
Water of Poppy   277
Water of Mint   296
Water of Marigold flowers   298
Water of Snails   294

FINIS.

Lightning Source UK Ltd.
Milton Keynes UK
UKHW030633280319
340058UK00006B/359/P